THE ARTHRITIS COOKBOOK

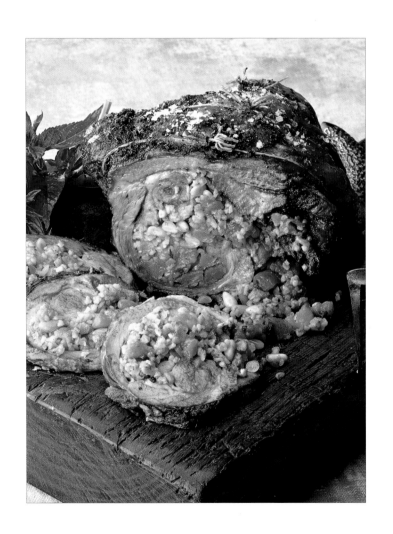

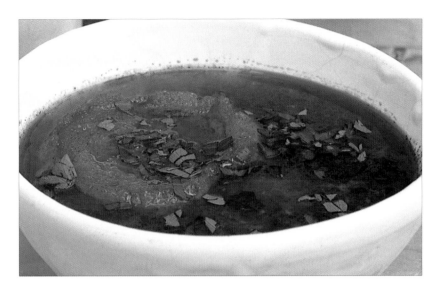

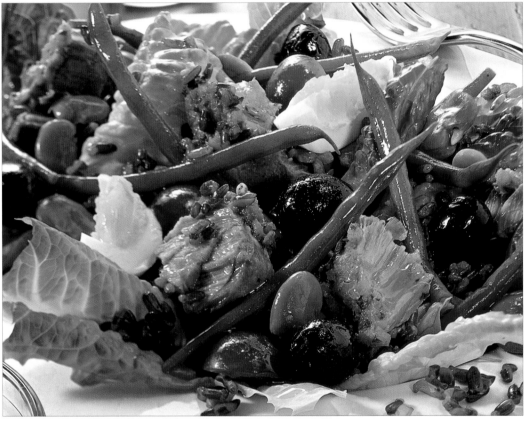

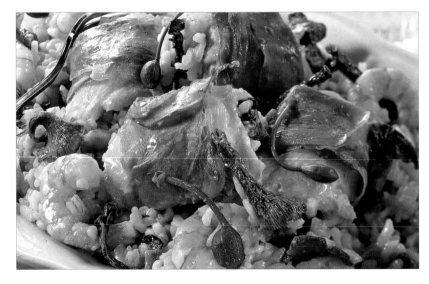

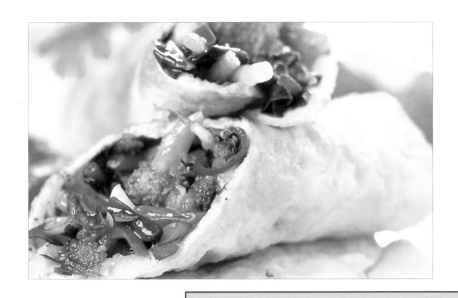

THE ARTHRITIS COOKBOOK

OVER 50 DELICIOUS AND HEALTHY RECIPES FOR PEOPLE WITH ARTHRITIS

MICHELLE BERRIEDALE-JOHNSON

LORENZ BOOKS

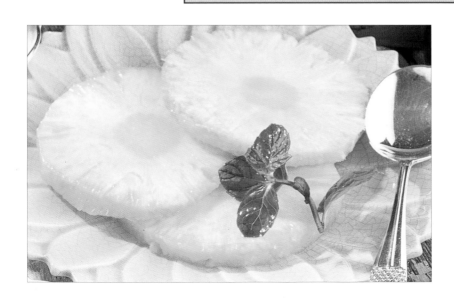

This edition published in 2000 by Lorenz Books

Lorenz Books is an imprint of
Anness Publishing Limited
Hermes House
88–89 Blackfriars Road
London SE1 8HA

This edition is distributed in Canada by Raincoast Books, 8680 Cambie Street,
Vancouver, British Columbia V6P 6MQ

A CIP catalogue record for this book is available from the British Library.

Publisher: Joanna Lorenz
Executive Editor: Linda Fraser
Project Editor: Rebecca Clunes
Designer: Ian Sandom
Recipes by: Carla Capalbo, Lesley Chamberlain, Jacqueline Clark, Carole Clements,
Andi Clevely, Roz Denny, Joanna Farrow, Nicola Graimes, Christine Ingram,
Peter Jordan, Lesley Mackley, Sally Mansfield, Sallie Morris, Katherine Richmond,
Liz Trigg, Lara Washburn, Stephen Wheeler, Elizabeth Wolf-Cohen, Jeni Wright
Photographer for introduction section: Janine Hosegood
Photographers for recipes: James Duncan, John Freeman, Ian Garlick, Michelle Garrett,
Amanda Heywood, Dave Jordan, Dave King, William Lingwood, Michael Michaels,
Thomas Odulate, Sam Stowell
Typesetter: Diane Pullen
Nutritional Analysis: Clare Brain
Indexer: Hilary Bird

1 3 5 7 9 10 8 6 4 2

NOTES

For all recipes, quantities are given in both metric and imperial measures and, where
appropriate, measures are also given in standard cups and spoons. Follow one set, but
not a mixture, because they are not interchangeable.

Standard spoon and cup measures are level.

1 tsp = 5ml, 1 tbsp = 15ml, 1 cup = 250ml/8fl oz

Australian standard tablespoons are 20ml. Australian readers should use 3 tsp in place
of 1 tbsp for measuring small quantities of gelatine, cornflour, salt, etc.

Medium eggs are used unless otherwise stated.

NSP is the new term for fibre. It stands for Non-Starch Polysaccharides. Using older
methods of analysis, the recommended fibre intake was 20g per person per day. Using
the new method this figure becomes about 11–13g.

Portion sizes: The recipes in this book are generally for four people. They can be halved
or quartered, depending on the number of servings required.

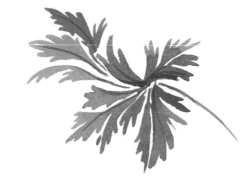

CONTENTS

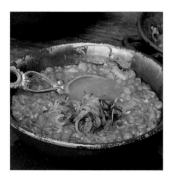

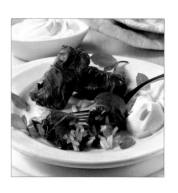

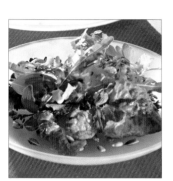

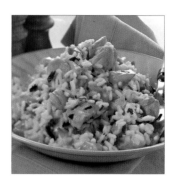

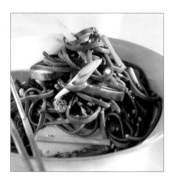

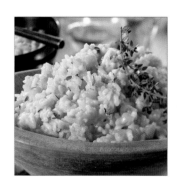

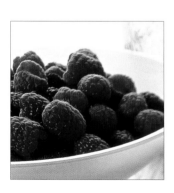

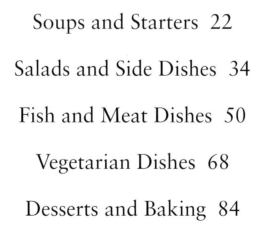

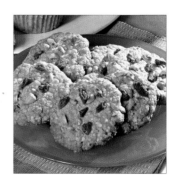

INTRODUCTION

Arthritis is a condition that can affect any of the joints, but is especially prevalent in the load-bearing or particularly hard-working areas, such as the knees, hips, ankles, wrists and hands. In the Western world it is estimated that up to half the population will suffer from an arthritic disorder of the joints at some point in their lives, and that many of these people will be severely troubled by constant pain, stiffness and disability. This is obviously a depressing prospect.

Arthritis cannot be treated as a single disease. There are at least six common forms and up to 100 lesser known types, excluding the rheumatic ailments that are often confused with arthritis. Although it is just as painful as arthritis, rheumatism (including fibrositis/fibromyalgia, bursitis, frozen shoulder and aching neck) is a less serious condition affecting muscles, ligaments and tendons.

Human joints are extremely complex and flexible structures, but they require "good maintenance" for efficient, long-term function. It is when a joint is damaged that arthritis can set in. Damage can be caused by a wide variety of incidents: trauma or accident, abnormal stress, maybe even viral infection or an inflammation. Confusingly, damage may not always lead to arthritis and, as yet, beyond a genetic predisposition, doctors have been unable to identify why some people develop arthritis-related conditions while others do not.

THE STRUCTURE OF A JOINT

A joint is made up of two connecting bones, separated and cushioned by cartilage. Cartilage is water-filled, spongy tissue with no blood vessels and no nerve endings, so cartilage itself never hurts. The joint is held together by a tubular structure attached to the ends of the bones. This is lined with a synovial membrane and lubricated by synovial fluid, which allows the moving parts to rub against each other with minimum friction. The joint is stabilized by muscles, ligaments and tendons on both its inside and outside.

CHANGES IN A DAMAGED AND ARTHRITIC JOINT

The protective cartilage is vital to the proper functioning of the joint. If the cartilage is damaged in any way it is less efficient as the cushion separating the bones.

When the cartilage ceases to perform its cushioning function properly there are several consequences. Initially there appears to be some water loss, after which the cartilage thickens and then softens. Small rips may appear and gradually deepen into tears, which may extend as far as the bone. The bone ends may be damaged or the joint capsule and synovial membrane may become damaged or inflamed. The surrounding tendons and ligaments may also be strained. Eventually, the bone attempts to repair the damage by forming bone spurs, and these stretch the sensitive membrane covering the bone to visibly deform the joints, causing further strain on the surrounding membranes and muscles. The synovial lining, fluid and capsule become inflamed and the joint stiffens.

Although the cartilage has no feeling, the other parts of the joint, including the bone, are very pain sensitive. Increasing pain and stiffness lead to immobility, and experience shows that immobility only makes the condition worse. This explains why most arthritis sufferers find their condition more painful in the morning after lying still all night, than later in the day after moving around.

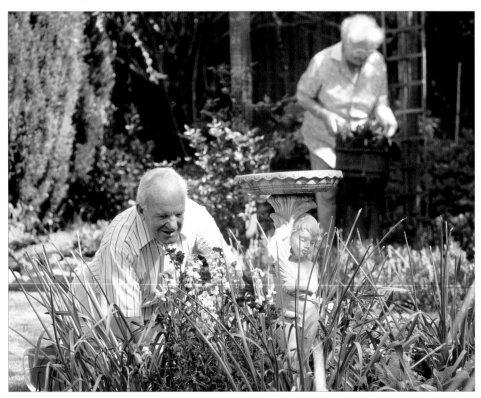

Left: Osteoarthritis often occurs in the joints that bear the most stress. Keen gardeners may find arthritis particularly painful in their knees, due to long hours of weeding.

Right: Arthritis can affect people of any age, even children. Juvenile arthritis can be particularly distressing, but the good news is that most children outgrow the condition, with no long-term effects.

TYPES OF ARTHRITIS

Although arthritis can take many different forms, the basic joint problem is the same for each type.

OSTEOARTHRITIS

This is the most common form of arthritis, usually associated with increasing age and degeneration. It is also more common in women. Osteoarthritis often occurs in a joint that has been injured or stressed, particularly those joints that do the most work – fingers and thumbs, wrists, knees, hips, ankles and toes. Bony spurs form around the joints and, along with inflammation, make movement difficult and painful.

Progressive joint deterioration can create secondary problems, such as carpal tunnel syndrome, which occurs when arthritis of the wrist causes nerves to be pinched. Not only does this produce pain, but also weakness and loss of control in the hands. Arthritis of the neck can cause severe headaches. Arthritis of the spine can cause radiating pain into the arm or leg (known as sciatica), or injury to the spinal column or the nerves within the spinal canal.

RHEUMATOID ARTHRITIS

This condition tends to occur in younger people. It is very dramatic and unpredictable and has been known to disappear as suddenly as it appears. It causes inflammation, pain, swelling and joint damage, especially in the hands and wrists, feet, knees and elbows. In severe cases rheumatoid arthritis can affect the internal organs – lungs, heart, liver, kidneys and lymph nodes.

Although no single cause has been found for rheumatoid arthritis, there is evidence to suggest that food allergies,

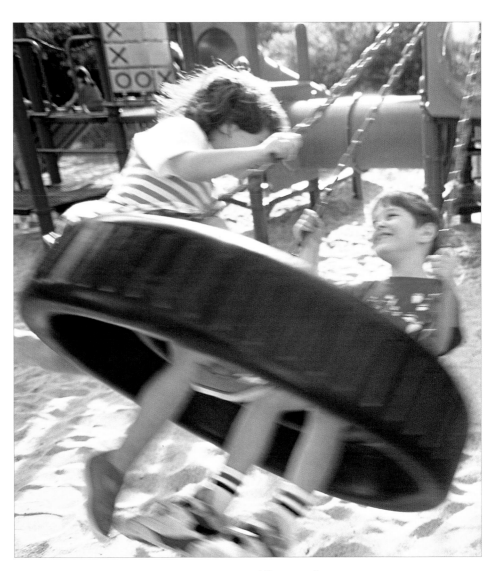

nutritional deficiencies and viral, parasitic and bacterial infections contribute to the condition.

ANKYLOSING SPONDILITIS

This is an inflammatory condition of the lower back, and it can spread both up and down the spine. It is most common in men.

JUVENILE ARTHRITIS

Symptoms include pain, fever, swelling and skin rash. The condition seems to improve over time, leaving the child with little serious joint damage.

PSORIATIC ARTHRITIS

A condition in which psoriasis (patches of raised, flaky and itching skin) and arthritis are combined.

VIRAL ARTHRITIS

This illness can follow a viral infection, whether or not the person already suffers from arthritis.

LUPUS ERYTHEMATOSUS

This condition causes inflammation of the connective tissue. Symptoms are influenza-like, including aching muscles and joints, fever and fatigue.

GOUT

This is caused by an excess of uric acid in the system. The acid crystals are deposited around joints and tendons, causing inflammation and pain. It can usually be controlled by drugs and by avoiding purines (substances rich in uric acid), which are found in liver, kidneys, shellfish, sardines, anchovies and beer.

Treating Arthritis

Conventional medicine, on the whole, does not accept a link between food and arthritis. However, there is evidence to suggest that food intolerance and micro-nutrition (essential vitamins, minerals and trace elements) may play a significant role, especially in cases of rheumatoid arthritis.

CONVENTIONAL TREATMENT

Despite the fact that many people are disabled by the various forms of arthritis, medical science can offer no cure. Treatment therefore falls into four areas.

• **Minimizing stress on affected joints** Patients are often advised to lose weight. Although no one is quite sure why, it would appear that being overweight can negatively affect joints, including those that are not weight-bearing (fingers and wrists).

• **Keeping affected joints mobile** Regular, gentle exercise and physiotherapy will keep joints as supple as possible.

• **Reducing the pain of arthritis** Various pain-relieving drugs are used, normally corticosteroids and non-steroidal anti-inflammatory drugs (NSAIDs). Although they may relieve at least some of the inflammation and pain, they do nothing to reverse, or even slow down, the progress of the disease. These drugs can have serious side effects. Even short-term use of steroids can cause weight gain, the one thing that arthritics do not want. Long-term use can cause brittle bone disease or osteoporosis, muscle wasting, skin eruptions and damage, poor wound healing, fluid retention, eye disorders, nutritional deficiencies, even mental disturbance. NSAIDs most frequently cause stomach ulceration.

• **Clearing up infections** Some forms of arthritis (for example, certain cases of rheumatoid arthritis) seem to be set off by bacteria, such as salmonella, campylobacter or yersinai. Joint pains can linger for months or years. In such cases antibiotic treatment may be useful.

ALTERNATIVE TREATMENT

There are occasional cases where dramatic results are achieved by the exclusion or inclusion of one particular food in the diet. However, most people will find that a combined approach, following some of the suggestions below, will result in an improvement in their symptoms, if not a total cure.

• **Dietary manipulation of inflammation** This means eating foods that are most likely to reduce inflammation in the joints.

• **Vitamin and mineral supplementation** Eating a diet rich in the vitamins and minerals needed to minimize the damage caused by arthritis, while taking supplements to counteract possible deficiencies.

• **Exclusion diet** Pinpointing and then removing a particular food, such as wheat or tomatoes, that triggers arthritis or makes the symptoms worse.

• **Weight control** Following a diet to keep body weight down.

OTHER CAUSES

As with most other illnesses, stress seems to make arthritis worse and prevents healing, so minimizing stress is an important part of both complementary and conventional forms of treatment.

There is also some evidence to suggest that, although imbalance in the gut flora (an overgrowth of the yeast *candida albicans*) will not actually cause arthritis, it may well make the symptoms worse.

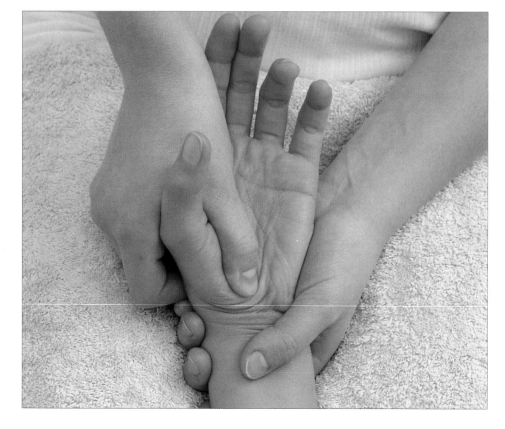

Left: A doctor will often recommend physiotherapy for joints affected by arthritis, as immobility only aggravates the condition. A gentle massage will help to keep your joints as supple as possible.

LOSING WEIGHT

This is a universal recommendation in the treatment of all types of arthritis, and so you need to make it a priority when you are planning your diet. Many of the dietary recommendations for weight loss will also help to increase antioxidant levels and reduce inflammation of the joints.

Most dieticians recommend a gradual weight loss, increasing your intake of vegetables, pulses and some grains, while reducing the fat content of your diet, especially animal fats. In addition, reducing the amount of sugar and refined white flour in a diet will usually put most people well on the way to losing the required amount of weight.

Reducing the intake of sugar and refined flours does not cut out all prospect of desserts, cake or biscuits. Fruits such as dates, prunes, raisins, apples and pears are excellent for sweetening puddings and cakes, and there are many flours, from wholemeal (wheat) flour to rice or chick-pea flour, which are just as versatile as ordinary white flour.

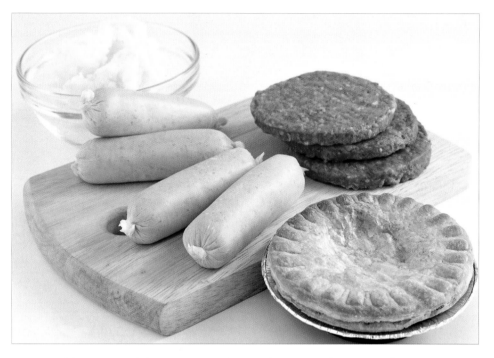

Above: Fatty foods, especially meat and cooking fats derived from animals, can increase the swelling and pain in arthritic joints.

NEW COOKING METHODS

Adjusting the way food is cooked is one easy way to reduce the use of cooking oils.

Deep-fried foods should be banned from the menu. Occasional shallow frying in a little olive oil with a tablespoon of water added (to prevent the oil overheating) is fine, but it is amazing how often grilling, roasting, poaching, steaming, baking or simmering can be used instead of frying. If you are still eating meat, grill sausages, bacon, fish fingers and burgers. Eggs taste delicious poached. Potatoes can be baked or steamed, or, if you are really desperate for chips, treat yourself to the occasional helping of oven chips, which are much lower in fat. Casseroles – for which ingredients are usually first fried in oil – often taste just as good if this step is omitted. Simply combine all the ingredients and cook the whole dish a little longer at a lower temperature, so as to allow the flavours to mature.

Vegetables are much better steamed than boiled as this cooking method does not allow so many nutrients to leach out and the vegetables have less opportunity to overcook.

Sweating is another good cooking method. This needs only a very small amount of oil (about 15ml/1 tbsp) with 15ml/1 tbsp water. Put the vegetables, oil and water into a saucepan with a tight-fitting lid and cook them slowly in their own juices. You will lose very few of the nutrients, apart from some Vitamin C, which will be lost no matter what your cooking method.

EATING LESS MEAT

Vegetarians seem to have less trouble with arthritis than people who eat meat, so there is an argument for trying to reduce the overall consumption of meat. If the idea of a totally vegetarian meal does not appeal, there are a number of meat substitutes that taste fine. Quorn and TVP (textured vegetable protein) have a texture similar to chicken and, like plain beancurd (tofu), are relatively tasteless but absorb other flavours well. They can all be used with marinades, in curries, casseroles or stews with plenty of herbs and full-flavoured vegetables. Beancurd is also available smoked and ready marinated and can be used in stir-fries, risottos, pilaffs, bean dishes and salads with a good strong dressing (this is a good opportunity to use some inflammation-reducing oil).

Include some totally vegetarian meals in your weekly diet. A good selection of vegetables, roasted with some herbs and a few nuts, makes an excellent and very easy dish. Dishes made with beans, nuts, seeds, herbs, spices and seaweeds (which are now fairly easy to obtain and have a wonderful flavour) are exciting, filling, healthy – and not fattening!

Reducing Inflammation

Inflammation is the body's way of bringing extra blood, with all its healing nutrients, to an injured area of the body. In the case of arthritis the extra blood, far from healing the injury, creates extra heat and swelling which merely add to the stiffness and soreness of the joint.

The inflammation of the joints that is associated with arthritis can be triggered, often on an ongoing basis, by damage to some part of the joint. Another possible cause is a malfunction in the body's mechanisms for triggering inflammation.

Various foods, especially fats, can influence the inflammatory process in either a negative or a positive way. This is because the chemicals (prostaglandins) that control inflammation are derived from fats in the body. Prostaglandin E2 is the chemical that sparks off the inflammation; it is derived mainly from the fats found in meat and cooking oils. Prostaglandins E1 and E3 act in quite the opposite way, to block swelling and reduce the pain and heat. Prostaglandin E1 is derived from gamma linolenic acid (GLA) found only in a few seed oils – borage, evening primrose, blackcurrant and hemp/linseed. Prostaglandin E3 is derived from alpha linolenic acid (ALA) and is found in green leafy vegetables, rape seed oil, wheat germ oil and oily fish.

Although these fats do not work in exactly the same way for everyone, decreasing the amount of fat in the diet from animal sources and cooking oils and increasing plant foods, seeds and oily fish may help to reduce inflammation without the unwanted side effects caused by drugs. This is one of the reasons why many arthritics find a vegetarian or vegan diet, that is free of animal products, helpful.

Gamma Linolenic Acid (GLA)

Eating more seeds and seed oils is the easiest way to increase GLA intake to make the inflammation-reducing prostaglandins. Evening primrose, borage and blackcurrant oils can all be taken as supplements, but hemp, or linseed, oil has to be taken as an oil and this unfortunately has an unpleasant taste. There is one seed oil

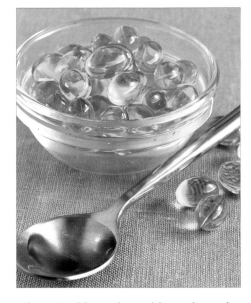

Above: Cod liver oil or cod liver oil capsules are an excellent way of boosting your intake of ALAs, which in turn will help to control the inflammation caused by arthritis.

blended by a Canadian, Professor Udo Erasmus, an acknowledged expert on the role of fats in the diet and in degenerative diseases such as arthritis. Known as Udo's Oil, it tastes pleasant enough to be used as a salad oil and, although expensive, it is an excellent way of boosting GLA intake.

Eating pumpkin, sunflower, sesame and linseeds will also help to boost your intake – they can be eaten as they are or added to almost any dish. Use the seeds whole, when they will have to be chewed well to release the oils, or process them briefly in a pestle and mortar, coffee grinder or a food processor to lightly grind them. Whole seeds can be lightly toasted under the grill to vary their flavour.

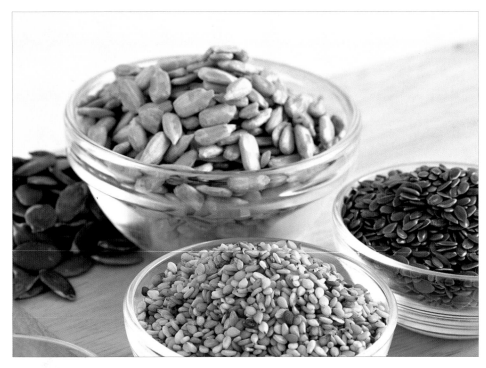

Left: Some seeds contain useful amounts of helpful GLAs. Try to use a handful of seeds in every meal. Clockwise from top: sunflower seeds, linseed, sesame seeds and pumpkin seeds.

ALPHA LINOLENIC ACID (ALA)

Reducing your intake of animal fats usually means eating more fresh fruits and vegetables – which boosts consumption of alpha linolenic acid (ALA), used to manufacture prostaglandin E3. Wheatgerm oil supplement will further boost alpha linolenic acid intake – but this is not suitable for those excluding wheat from the diet. Eating oily fish is also a good way to increase ALA in the diet. The term "oily" fish may sound rather unattractive, but, in fact, sardines, anchovies, mackerel, salmon, herrings, kippers and whitebait are one of the tastiest types of seafood. Most can be bought in a form where you do not have to fiddle with fish bones or skin, and some types can be eaten whole. Pre-prepared fish can be bought fresh, frozen or canned. As well as using oily fish as the main dish, add them in small quantities to salads and rice, bean or vegetable dishes. Try using anchovies to season some of your dishes instead of salt. As well as boosting your ALA levels, you will be reducing your sodium intake and helping to control high blood pressure.

GINGER

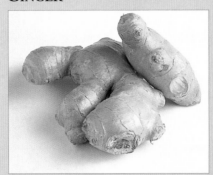

This spice has been used for centuries in traditional Indian Ayurvedic medicine as an anti-inflammatory food. It blocks the enzymes that make the inflammation-producing prostaglandins. Ginger does not work for everyone, but a dose of 1–2 grams of ground ginger or a 25g/2oz knob of fresh ginger, peeled and grated, taken daily over a period of 3–4 months, appears to produce very positive results in the symptoms of over half the people who try it.

If you like ginger, you can consume it as a drink (there are a number of herbal teas with ginger), in ginger wine or as a confection, coated in chocolate. Ground ginger can be used in puddings, cakes and biscuits, and fresh root ginger is delicious in a wide variety of savoury dishes. You can even eat crystallized or stem ginger in ice cream.

Below: Oily fish are one of the best foods for reducing inflammation. It is, however, sometimes tricky to know which fish belong to this category. Tuna, for instance, is not an oily fish. Clockwise from bottom left: tuna steak, mackerel, herring, salmon steak.

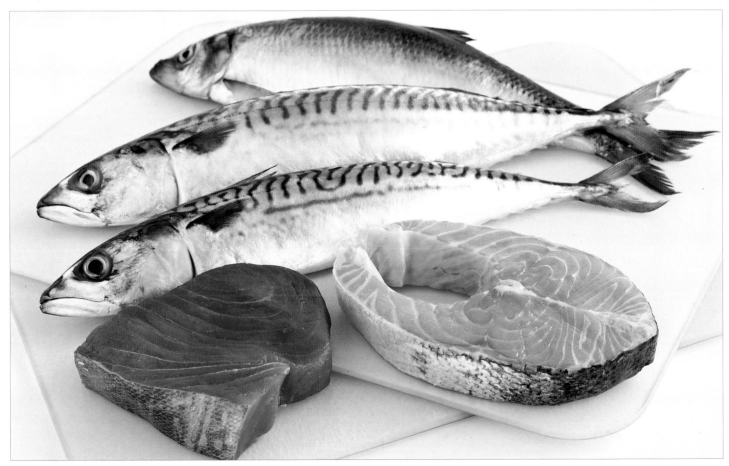

INCREASING VITAMINS AND MINERALS

Even with a balanced and healthy diet, "micro-nutrient malnutrition" may occur, especially as people grow older. This can either be the result of a deficiency of vitamins and minerals in the diet, or of the body's failure to absorb these substances properly from food.

If bones and joints are not receiving enough of the vitamins and minerals needed to maintain them, they are more likely to degenerate. Taking a "broad spectrum" supplement or a multi-vitamin and mineral supplement is helpful, but it may be worth consulting a nutritionist and having a blood test to assess whether the body is deficient in any specific mineral. Iron, zinc, copper, selenium and manganese are all important minerals for joint health, and their absorption can be impeded by consuming too much tea, coffee and bran. The traditional arthritis remedy of wearing a copper bracelet can be helpful, as small quantities of copper can be absorbed through the skin.

FREE RADICALS

Most people have heard of free radicals in connection with cancer; they are also relevant in arthritis. As oxygen is processed through the bloodstream and into the tissues, free radical chemicals (including hydrogen peroxide) are released. Although these free radicals are very unstable and only exist for 1–2 seconds, in this short time they can cause all kinds of damage in the body including taking hydrogen electrons from molecules in body tissues and damaging the tissues in the process. Antioxidants neutralize these free radicals by donating extra hydrogen electrons to them before they can take them from the body tissues. You should eat plenty of foods rich in antioxidants: vitamins A, C, E and betacarotene are the best known of these nutrients, although lycopene (found in tomatoes), zinc and manganese are also important. Many flavonoids (the chemicals that give peppers and fruits such as blueberries, blackberries, cherries and lemons their colour) are also powerful antioxidants.

It is important that anyone with arthritis absorbs plenty of antioxidants, both by eating a diet rich in antioxidants and by taking a vitamin and mineral supplement. Ideally, these supplements should be taken under medical or nutritional supervision, so that they can be adapted to suit your particular needs.

VITAMIN A

Found in liver, especially fish liver oils, eggs, orange and yellow fruits, and green leafy vegetables, vitamin A should not be taken in excess, that is, in levels of over 10,000 IUs per day. A spoonful of that old favourite, cod liver oil, is the simple, if not the most pleasant, way of increasing Vitamin A intake. Alternatively, include chicken, calf's or lamb's liver in some dishes.

Left: Drinking too much tea and coffee may reduce the absorption of vital minerals, particularly iron. Naturally flavoured fruit teas are a good substitute, and contain almost no calories.

A little chicken liver can be added to a meat stew without changing the flavour too much. However, as arthritis sufferers should be trying to reduce meat consumption, it is better to eat a fairly regular supply of eggs and eat plenty of yellow and orange vegetables (carrots, yellow, orange and red peppers, and yellow squash) and fruits in salads and vegetable dishes.

VITAMIN C

This is found in most fresh fruits and vegetables but is easily destroyed by the cooking process. Eating more fresh, raw fruit and vegetables automatically increases vitamin C consumption. People who are avoiding citrus fruits or members of the solanacae family (potatoes, peppers, chillies, tomatoes, aubergines) as part of an exclusion diet will still find an abundance of other fresh fruits and vegetables that contain substantial quantities of vitamin C.

VITAMIN E

This is found in most vegetable oils (olive, corn and so on), nuts, seeds, avocados (which are also a rich source of vitamin C), peaches, broccoli, spinach and asparagus. The seeds and seed oils that are eaten as part of an anti-inflammatory diet will therefore have the additional benefit of providing a substantial amount of vitamin E.

SELENIUM

Grains and nuts are sources of selenium, but their precise content varies according to the soil in which they were grown. Selenium interacts with vitamin E, making both of these nutrients more powerful. Brazil nuts, grains and pulses (especially lentils), mung beans and red kidney beans are good for boosting the levels in the diet. Fish is also a good source of selenium.

BETACAROTENE

This is the best known of over 600 carotenoids, which are the plant pigments that give yellow, orange and

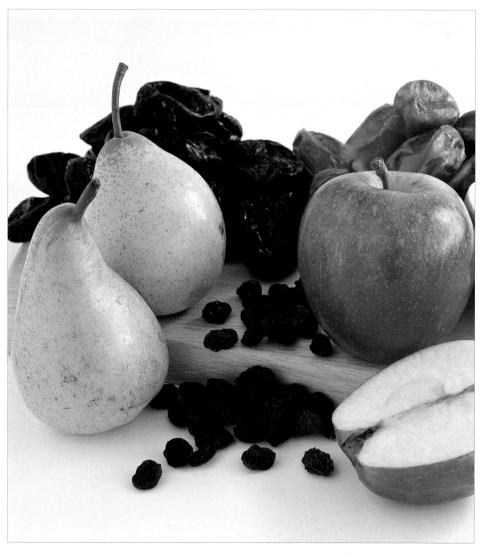

Above: Fruit is an excellent natural sweetener and can be used both fresh and dried. It also provides useful amounts of vitamin C and other trace elements.

Right: Supplements can ensure you receive the trace elements that may be missing, and are a useful source of antioxidants.

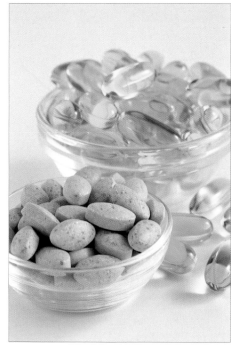

red fruits their colour. Scientists are greatly interested in carotenoids, which they suspect may be even more powerful antioxidants than the established vitamins A, C and E. Like many of the carotenoids, betacarotene can be converted by the body into vitamin A. Betacarotene is to be found in carrots, apricots, cantaloupe melon, sweet potatoes, pumpkin, spinach, kale and parsley.

FOOD ALLERGIES

Although most conventional specialists dismiss food allergy as being a cause of arthritis, there is a growing body of evidence to suggest that it may be a trigger in a substantial number of cases of rheumatoid arthritis and, to a more limited extent, in other types of arthritis as well.

The amount of the allergic food that is needed to trigger a reaction, the strength of the reaction itself and the improvement that can be achieved by excluding the food from the diet will all vary according to the individual. One sufferer's symptoms may disappear completely when they cut out the relevant food but return if they eat the smallest amount of the allergen. Another person may find that their condition improves to some extent if they cut down on a certain food, but it does not improve further if they cut the food out entirely. It is important that each person experiments with his or her own diet and is not put off by the experiences of other people.

Of course, not everyone will find that changing their diet will cure, or even improve, their arthritis. However, most people will benefit from eating a healthier, balanced diet and most arthritics, unless they are very slim, will probably benefit from losing some weight. There are few statistics, but it would appear that up to 40 per cent of arthritis sufferers (especially those with rheumatoid arthritis) may benefit to some extent by improving their diet. Of that 40 per cent, a small number will find themselves miraculously cured of the condition.

POTENTIALLY ALLERGIC FOODS

There is no food that is guaranteed not to cause an allergic reaction. Every food can provoke an allergy in someone, and it is perfectly possible that the allergy may show itself as arthritis. To complicate the issue, people can have an allergy to more than one food. So, to test properly for an allergic reaction, you need to try all foods, alone and together. Certain families of foods seem to be most frequently involved, however.

- Dairy products such as milk, cheese, cream, butter and yogurt.
- Vegetables from the deadly nightshade or solanacae family such as red, green and yellow peppers, potatoes, tomatoes, tobacco, chillies and aubergines.
- Citrus fruits, especially orange juice.
- Wheat and all wheat derivatives.

CANDIDA

If candida (yeast overgrowth in your system) is a problem then a two-pronged strategy is usual: treatment with anti-fungal medication and a diet excluding sugar and all fermented foods, starving the yeast of nourishment.

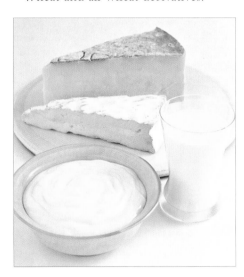

Above, clockwise from top: Dairy products include: Cheddar cheese, cow's milk, yogurt made from cow's milk, Brie.

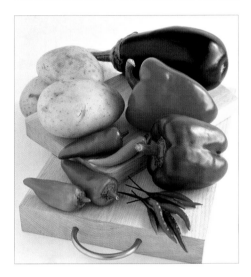

Above, clockwise from top: The solanacae family includes aubergine, red and green peppers, chillies, potatoes.

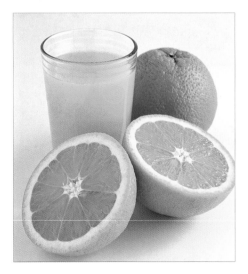

Above: Citrus fruits, and especially oranges and orange juice, can cause a severe allergic reaction in some people.

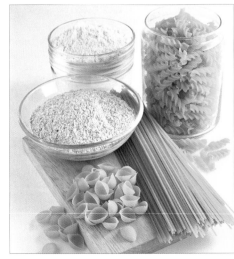

Above: Flour and pasta both contain wheat and should therefore be avoided by people following a wheat-free diet.

EXCLUSION DIETS

There is no guarantee that a food allergy has caused or worsened an individual case of arthritis; however, if it has, there are substantial benefits in altering the diet to exclude those foods that trigger the arthritis. They include reduced pain, improved mobility, less joint deterioration, reduced use of drugs and fewer side effects. For a few people, the effects are so positive as to amount to a cure. For most arthritics, excluding foods that their bodies cannot tolerate will not rid them of their arthritis, but it may improve their condition sufficiently to be worth the effort of excluding those foods. Also, if a food upsets the body enough to aggravate arthritis, it may be damaging to your health in other respects, so that excluding it, or at least reducing the amount eaten, will probably be good for your general health.

Before embarking on an exlusion diet, a nutritionist should be consulted by people on a lot of medication; who have health problems in addition to arthritis; who are very young or old; and anyone who is pregnant. A diet that excludes more than one group of foods (dairy products, citrus fruits, wheat and so on) should never be followed in such cases, except under medical supervision.

There are two methods of pinpointing the troublesome food: an allergy test and keeping a food diary.

ALLERGY TESTS

These vary in type and cost, from inexpensive tests offered by healthfood shops (which test for the basic six potential allergens) to a thorough blood analysis covering 100–200 foods and offering back-up information and advice. If you cannot face working through a strict exclusion diet for each of the possible groups of potentially allergic foods, an allergy test may be a worthwhile shortcut. The result still has to be verified by excluding the food from the diet for a period of time.

However, be cautious when reading the test results. If a test records a reaction to a very large number of foods, the advice of a dietician or nutritionist should be taken before excluding them from the diet. More harm than good results from a starvation diet. If there is a genuine bad reaction to a number of foods, professional nutritional guidance must be taken to work through the problem and find a balanced solution.

KEEPING A FOOD DIARY

A food diary will instil the habit of really thinking about all foods that are eaten. It should be kept for a couple of weeks. Note down everything eaten in the day, from licking the marmalade spoon after breakfast to finishing off the children's lunch. The diary must include notes on the arthritis condition – when it is worse or slightly better. There should be least five entries a day for both food and condition.

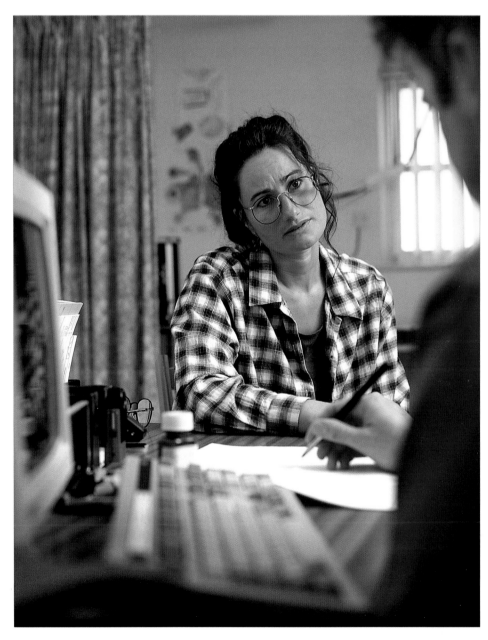

Above: It is a good idea to talk to your doctor or a nutritionist before embarking on an exclusion diet. He or she will be able to help you plan a diet so that you do not miss out on any essential food group.

DISCOVERING THE CULPRIT

After keeping a detailed food diary for a week or so, some kind of pattern may start to emerge. For example, do you always feel worse 30 minutes after a large glass of fresh orange juice for breakfast? The next step, and the only foolproof way to discover whether a food is having an adverse effect, is to exclude it from your diet for a period of at least one month. You will need to be patient when trying to pinpoint troublesome foods as the process may take several months.

EMBARKING ON AN EXCLUSION DIET

The suspect food family is most likely one of the four usually associated with arthritis – dairy products, citrus fruit, wheat and the solanacae family of vegetables. The food that you suspect you may be allergic to must be rigorously excluded from the diet for at least two weeks, preferably one month. It takes a surprisingly long time for the food to work its way out of the body completely and anyone genuinely sensitive to the food will react to the tiniest trace in the system.

It is relatively easy to exclude some foods from your diet, such as citrus fruits, as it is usually easy to identify them or dishes in which they have been used. It is far more difficult with the other three groups, however, as tomatoes, potatoes, dairy products and wheat products and their derivatives are used in almost every kind of ready-made food.

UNDERSTANDING LABELS

Although it is time-consuming, try to read every food label carefully to ensure that the product does not contain even a trace of the excluded food. To do this efficiently it is necessary to know all the names under which that product may appear on a label. For example, whey and casein are both constituents of milk and modified starch is made from wheat.

FOODS TO AVOID

These lists show some of the products and ingredients that are not necessarily instantly identified as a source of the foods to be excluded. This is extensive enough to highlight the problem – many more individual items could be added.

WHEAT
Foods
Couscous
Curry powder
Farina
Instant hot drinks (such as coffee, tea, chocolate)
Semolina
Soy sauce (except wheat-free tamari)
White pepper in restaurants (can be adulterated with flour)
Ingredients
Cereal filler
Modified starch
Monosodium glutamate
Rusk
Check labels of following:
Chinese sauces
Horseradish creams
Ketchups
Mustards
Prepared meats
Salad dressings
Sauces
Sausages
Seasoning mixes
Soups
Sweets (confectionery)

SOLANACAE
Aubergines
Bell peppers
Chilli peppers
Potatoes
Tomatoes
Spices
Cayenne pepper
Chilli powder
Curry powder
Paprika

DAIRY
Foods
Batter
Butter
Buttermilk
Cheese (including cream, curd and cottage cheeses)
Cream (double, whipping and single)
Créme fraîche
Ghee
Skimmed milk powder
Synthetic cream
Yogurt
Ingredients
Animal fats
Casein
Caseinates
Hydrolysed casein or whey
Lactose
Milk solids
Non-milk fat solids
Whey
Whey protein or sugar
Check labels of following:
Chocolate
Low-fat spreads
Vegetable fats

CITRUS FRUIT
Clementines
Grapefruit
Lemons
Limes
Mandarins
Mineolas
Oranges
Satsumas
Tangelos
Tangerines
Ugli fruits

The number of ready-made dishes that are suitable for people on an exclusion diet is small, although there are a growing number of companies producing foods without dairy products, wheat or other individual ingredients.

ALTERNATIVE INGREDIENTS

It has become fairly easy to find alternatives to some of the basic ingredients that are commonly excluded.

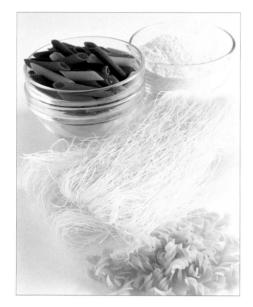

Above: There is now a wide range of non-wheat flours, noodles and pastas.

WHEAT-FREE DIET

Although the number of companies making flour, breads, pastas, pizzas, cake and biscuits without wheat is increasing all the time, they are still relatively few and the products are comparatively expensive. Potato flour or cornflour can be used for thickening soups, sauces and similar dishes, and bread, cakes and biscuits can be made using proprietary wheat-free flours, chick-pea flour or a combination of rice flour and ground oats.

DAIRY-FREE DIET

This means a diet free from cow's milk and all its products, not milk from sheep, goats or other animals.

Goat, sheep, soya or oat milk can be used instead of cow's milk for most savoury dishes, and there are dozens of different soya milks to choose from. For sweet dishes, both rice milk and coconut milk make good alternatives. There are a number of dairy-free spreads (check the ingredients list carefully) that can be substituted for

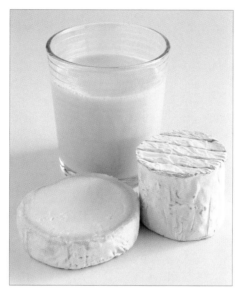

Above: Soya milk and goat's cheese are useful alternatives to dairy products.

butter, both on bread and for cooking or baking. There is also an increasing range of soya, sheep's milk and goat's milk yogurts and even ice creams. Cheese is a serious problem, as the food industry has still not managed to come up with a cheese substitute that tastes anything remotely like cheese, although there are a couple of soya "cheese" spreads which are perfectly harmless, if not terribly exciting.

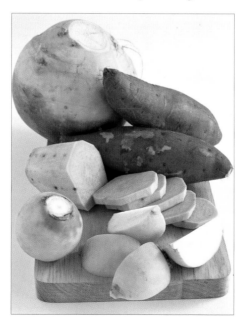

Above: Introduce hearty root vegetables such as swede, sweet potato and turnip.

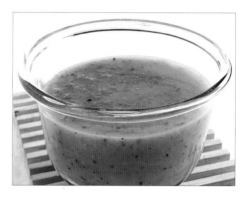

Above: A thick stock can be used instead of tomatoes in many recipes.

SOLANACAE-FREE DIET

This diet excludes potatoes, tomatoes, peppers, chillies and aubergines. There are a number of root vegetables that can be used instead of potatoes in many recipes, such as sweet potatoes, celeriac, Jerusalem artichokes, parsnips, swedes and carrots; firm squashes are also a useful alternative.

Tomatoes are the most difficult item to replace in this family, as there is really no satisfactory substitute for their sweet, acidic flavour and their juice. Use lots of chopped onions and plenty of herbs with a little thick and well-flavoured stock instead of tomatoes in recipes that rely on their juice.

Peppers, chillies and aubergines can be avoided fairly easily. The hot flavour of chilli can be replaced with black or white pepper. Remember, that cayenne pepper is a form of dried chillies and paprika is made from peppers.

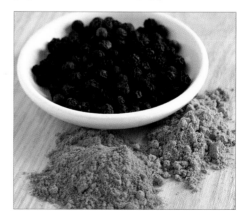

Above: Replace chillies with spices such as peppercorns, ground turmeric or ginger.

NO IMPROVEMENT?

A month on an exclusion diet may not yield any improvement in the arthritis. This may be because the wrong food group has been excluded. In that case, try again with another of the food groups. By working through all four of the food families, each will be eliminated in turn; it may be that this diet does not make any difference to the arthritis and that food group is genuinely not implicated in this case. Alternatively, the problem food may not have been located, or there could be more than one food causing the problem. There are a number of therapists who have had great success with specific diets which eliminate more than one type of food. For example, one American therapist, himself an ex-arthritic, recommends a diet regime including only seafood, vegetables and rice.

FOOD FASTS

If you have not had positive results after excluding the initial four food families, but still feel that food could be implicated, you might like to consider a food fast. On a four to five day fast, nothing but distilled water is consumed. If some food or drink is implicated, it will be excluded automatically during the fast and there should be an improvement. If there is a beneficial result, serious food detective work has to be used to track down the food – or foods – that cause the problem. No one should embark on such a fast lightly. It should ONLY be done when the person has time off, with nothing very much to do, and under the supervision of a doctor, dietician or nutritionist. This applies especially to those who are not in general good health, are on medication or who are very young, old or pregnant. Apart from the fact that not eating for extended periods creates

Right: A food fast should only ever be undertaken when you have time on your hands because you may find yourself reacting badly and feeling quite ill.

a feeling of light-headedness or results in headaches, anyone who reacts badly to certain foods may find that their body takes the opportunity to "detoxify" itself. This process can be quite dramatic and, like an alcoholic or a drug addict who is suddenly deprived of their addictive substance, the person can suddenly feel quite ill.

USING FOOD TO CHALLENGE A POSITIVE RESULT

If the exclusion diet has produced positive results and the arthritis is improved, if only a little, it has to be confirmed that it was the exclusion of that food that helped, not some other side effect of the diet or a change in lifestyle. Therefore the body has to be "challenged" with the food.

Re-introduce the excluded food in a reasonable quantity for one week. There may be an immediate reaction, or a far more gradual one after a few days. Either way, this confirms that the food is causing a problem. It is then up to the individual to decide whether the improvement in condition was worth the disruption to diet and daily life. It might be worth continuing your investigations into the diet to see whether other foods could be involved and whether further improvement may be possible if those foods are avoided.

A varied diet is always a good thing, and, as you continue to experiment with alternative ways of cooking and eating, you may even find yourself enjoying food more and regarding the experience as an adventure.

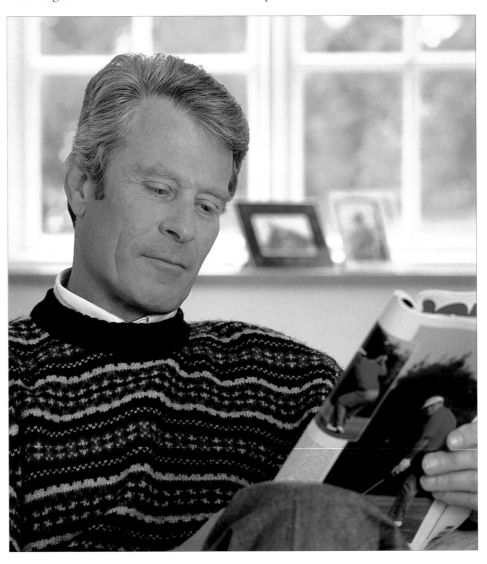

FOLLOWING A SPECIAL DIET

It is one thing knowing the theory, but quite another when it comes to putting it into practice, and this is particularly true of following a special diet. Try to be positive, focusing on different cooking methods and a variety of ingredients rather than on the foods to avoid.

A quick glance at all of these recommendations might give you the impression that you will lose weight very fast, as there may seem to be very little left that you are allowed to eat. However, a diet adjusted to help ease arthritis can include just as much variety as a standard diet. It may take a little extra effort, but there is no reason why the changes should not be included in the family eating pattern. As long as the changes are discreet, even fussy eaters will probably never notice. Adding new foods – especially when many of them are really tasty – is often easier than removing old favourites. In either case, involving the whole family in the diet makes catering easier and can turn into a culinary adventure for everyone.

Browse through a few cookbooks from a range of different cultures for inspiration. Try traditional dishes from India, China, Malaysia and Indonesia, for example, and you will be amazed at the number of fabulous dishes that are low in animal fats and high in the foods and nutrients you should be eating more of.

A FEW SIMPLE POINTS

• Use olive or sunflower oil for cooking rather than butter or lard.
• Try beancurd (tofu) or TVP/soya protein in a well-flavoured curry or stew instead of meat.
• Use soya, oat or rice milk in cooking rather than cow's milk.
• Cut down on chocolate, cakes and biscuits, and increase your intake of fresh fruit.
• Add a few seeds or nuts to savoury and sweet cooked dishes and to salads.
• Increase the number of raw vegetables that you eat.
• Try baking or steaming vegetables rather than frying or roasting them.

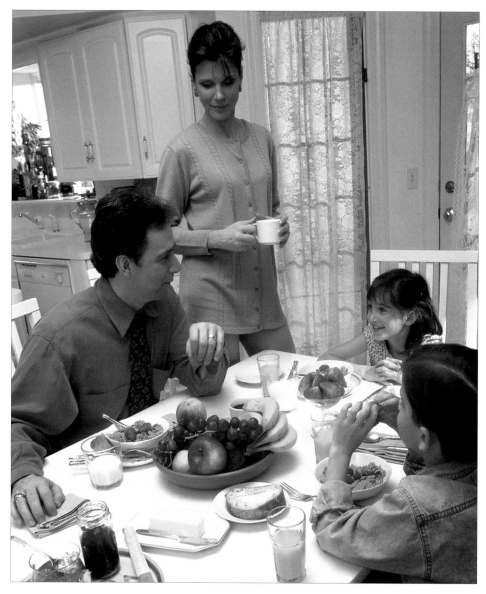

Above: A diet suitable for people with arthritis is low in fat and high in vitamins, and should be suitable for all members of the family. You will find it much easier to follow your diet if the rest of the family eat the same foods.

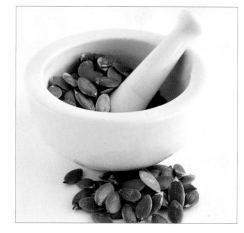

Right: Crushed pumpkin seeds can be used in a wide variety of dishes to increase your intake of GLAs. Try adding them to pastry or wholemeal scones, sprinkling them over salads or stirring them into casseroles or risotto.

KITCHEN IMPROVEMENTS

With arthritis there is a good chance that your hands, and indeed the rest of your body, are not as agile or as mobile as they once were. Although we would hope that changing your diet improves the condition, it is also a good idea to look around the kitchen for anything that could be changed to make cooking easier.

If your hands are stiff or weak, if you use a stick, find it difficult to stand for long, or have trouble bending, there are a number of relatively minor alterations that can be made to kitchen units and fixed appliances to make your life easier. There are also a few special gadgets that are not too expensive and can make quite a difference.

CUPBOARDS

If opening cupboard doors is difficult, take the doors off, leaving open shelves (very fashionable) or add curtains, which can be pulled across easily. Consider taking shelves out of base units to make space for sitting at the counter with your knees underneath or to store a trolley. If the work surfaces are too deep for you to reach the back wall comfortably, try adding a free-standing shallow storage shelf against the back wall. A rail along the front of the units provides extra support when getting around the kitchen and somewhere to hang a stick – as well as a dish towel. Many people prefer to cook sitting down so, if the units are too high, a small table can be ideal for sitting down to carry out some of the tasks involved in food preparation.

ELECTRICS

Rocker switches can be installed (this means changing just the fitment) and you can buy plugs with handles for all appliances that are much easier to pull out of sockets.

TAPS

Lever taps are easier to operate than the regular type. If you do not want to change the taps, lever tap-turners can be fitted on existing taps.

COOKERS AND MICROWAVES

A split-level cooker with an eye-level grill is very useful for people who cannot bend. Even better, a worktop combination microwave and convection cooker is very accessible. Appliances with a rocker door opener will be easier to use for anyone with weak hands. A cheaper alternative for a small family is a small microwave and a table-top oven or cooker. All these plug into a standard socket and are easy to use and clean. Table-top cookers get very hot, so care must be taken when using them. Multi-cookers, similar to electric frying pans, are also useful as they sit on a table. They can be used for boiling, stewing, roasting or baking, and some food can be served straight from the pan.

TROLLEYS

A trolley, ideally a fairly tall one, is invaluable in the kitchen for use as a table. It can also be pushed around as a walker-cum-trolley, and its handle provides somewhere for hanging a stick. Retail catalogues listing disabled equipment usually have a selection of reasonably priced, sturdy trolleys suitable for use in the kitchen.

Below: A small table can be ideal for chopping vegetables.

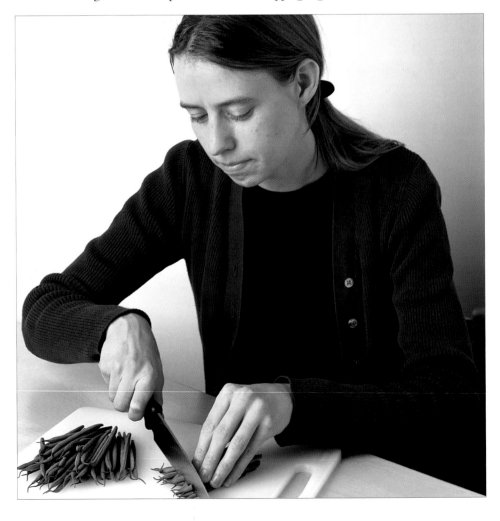

TONGS, KNIVES AND SCISSORS

A pair of long-handled tongs with insulated handles is invaluable for all kinds of tasks. Avoid using knives as far as possible, as it is all too easy to let them slip. Scissors can be used for many types of chopping jobs. Buy scissors with large chunky finger holds or that spring open automatically.

GRATERS, CAN OPENERS AND SCREWTOP OPENERS

Graters, especially the steady four-sided ones, are useful for many jobs. A plastic food mill, which grates by turning, is also handy. An electric can opener may be the answer for those with stiff hands, but a manual opener with chunky handles and an easy-to-grasp turning knob is less expensive. There are a selection of devices for removing tops from jars. Experiment in a gadget shop to find the one that you prefer.

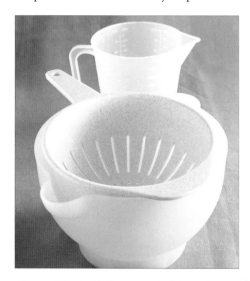

Above: Plastic kitchenware is lighter than metal and therefore easier to lift.

BOWLS AND MEASURING JUGS

Look for kitchen equipment made from lightweight plastic. Replace any ceramic mixing bowls, glass measuring jugs and metal colanders. If you are worried about the plastic bowl slipping when you are mixing, use a wet dish towel or a rubber mat (there are special mats called Dycem which are very good) to stop any movement.

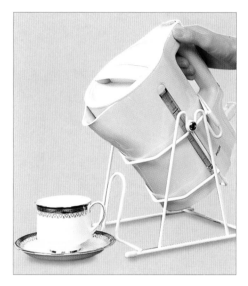

Above: A kettle tipper takes the weight of the water and also makes pouring safer.

KETTLES

A kettle that can be filled through the spout and that is neither too heavy nor too difficult to lift is essential – always test it before buying. Kettle tippers, which save you from having to lift the appliance for pouring, are available.

HANDLES

Choose cutlery and equipment with big, plump handles. If you do not want to buy new items, you can buy large plastic handles that fit over existing ones. Less elegant, but equally effective for cutlery, is a piece of rubber tubing taped firmly in place. Some specialist cutlery has handles that can be bent. The user can move them into the position they find most comfortable.

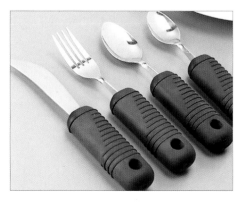

Above: Cutlery with big, chunky handles is easier to grip.

HELPING HANDS

A pair of magnetic pincers controlled by a lever on the end of a long handle is invaluable for picking up items when your reach is impaired. Helping hands are usually available from larger kitchen or hardware stores.

PROCESSORS, MIXERS AND LIQUIDIZERS

Small, hand-held appliances are easier to use than family-size models, most of which are heavy. Battery-powered cordless mixers are ideal.

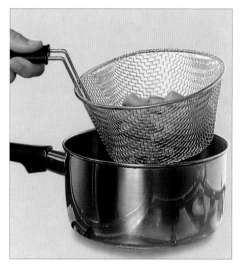

Above: A cooking basket will stop you having to lift a heavy pan of boiling water.

SAUCEPANS

Iron casseroles may be wonderful for long, slow cooking, but they are hard for even able-bodied cooks to lift. Look for good-quality, light pans with long handles. The handles must be big and easy to grasp as well as being well insulated. Twin-handled pans are ideal for people with weak hands.

Chose a non-stick pan that will be easy to clean. Cooking in a non-stick pan requires less fat, another important consideration for arthritis sufferers.

A stainless steel cooking basket is a useful investment as it allows you to remove and drain cooked vegetables without lifting a heavy pan of water. The pan can be emptied later when the water is cool.

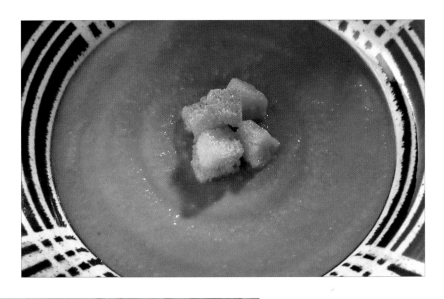

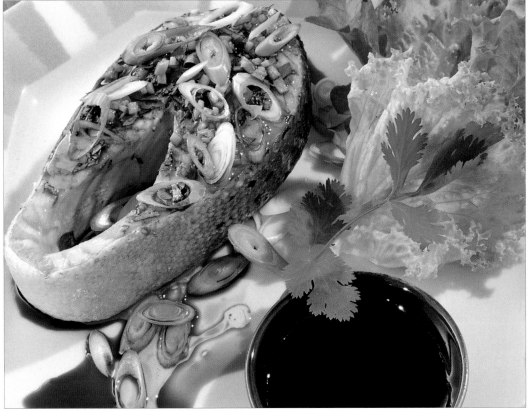

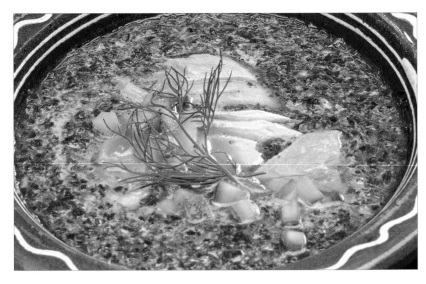

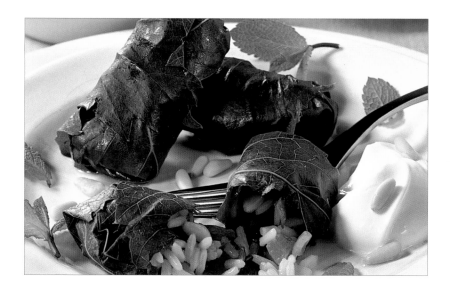

SOUPS AND STARTERS

Nutritious, easy to eat and easy to make, soups are excellent for people with arthritis. They can be cooked in one pot, puréed with a hand-held blender and drunk from a mug. Try one of the healthy starters and boost your GLA intake with Grilled Green Mussels with Cumin or experiment with Sizzling Salmon with Herbs. Remember that if your hands are stiff it is easier – and safer – to chop herbs, bacon and dried fruit with scissors than knives.

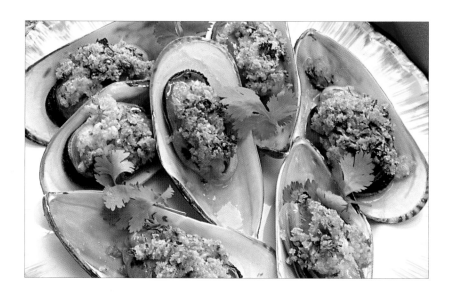

Fresh Pea Soup

This soup is a version of an old French recipe. Frozen peas are an excellent choice for those with arthritis: they are high in vitamin C and need no preparation.

INGREDIENTS

Serves 2

30ml/2 tbsp oil
2-3 shallots, finely chopped or 15ml/1 tbsp dried onion
400g/14oz/3 cups shelled fresh peas (from about 1.3kg/3lb garden peas) or thawed frozen peas
475ml/16fl oz/2 cups water
45ml/3 tbsp single cream, or omit if you are on a dairy-free diet
salt and ground black pepper
croûtons or crumbled crisp bacon, to garnish

1 Heat the oil in a flameproof casserole or saucepan. Add the shallots or dried onion and cook for about 3 minutes, stirring occasionally.

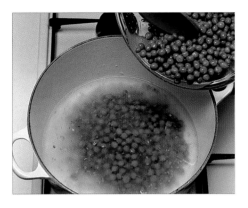

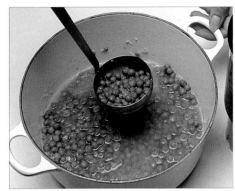

2 Add the peas and water. Cover the saucepan and allow the mixture to simmer for about 12 minutes if you are using young or frozen peas and up to 18 minutes for large or older peas, stirring occasionally.

3 When the peas are tender, ladle them into a blender or food processor with a little of the cooking liquid and process, in batches if necessary, until the mixture is smooth.

--- COOK'S TIP ---

If your hands are stiff and painful you can purée the soup in the pan with a hand-held blender and not strain it. The result won't be as smooth but will be just as tasty.

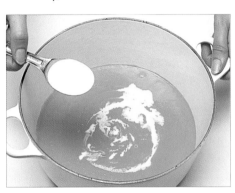

4 Strain the soup through a fine sieve back into the casserole or saucepan. Stir in the cream, if using, and heat the soup through without boiling. Season with salt and freshly ground black pepper to taste and serve hot, garnished with croûtons or bacon.

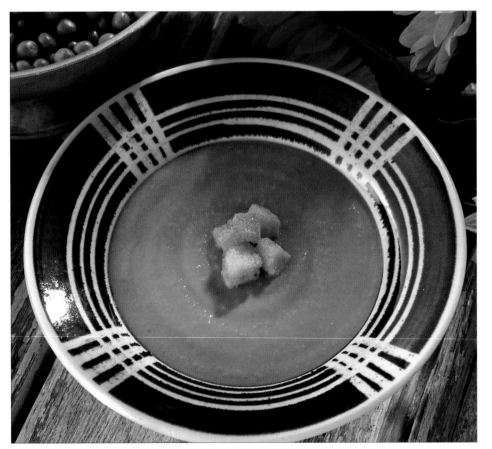

--- NUTRITION NOTES ---

Per portion:

Energy	309kcals/1266kJ
Fat, total	17.2g
saturated fat	4.6g
Protein	13.1g
Carbohydrate	27.0g
sugar, total	11.4g
Fibre – NSP	11.3g
Sodium	30.6mg

Asparagus Soup with Crab

This soup has a subtle flavour that is bound to impress. Asparagus is a good source of vitamin E.

INGREDIENTS

Serves 6

1.3kg/3lb fresh asparagus
30ml/2 tbsp olive oil
1.5 litres/2½ pints/6¼ cups vegetable
  stock
30ml/2 tbsp cornflour
45ml/3 tbsp single cream, or omit if
  you are on a dairy-free diet
salt and ground black pepper
175–200g/6–7oz white crab meat,
  to garnish

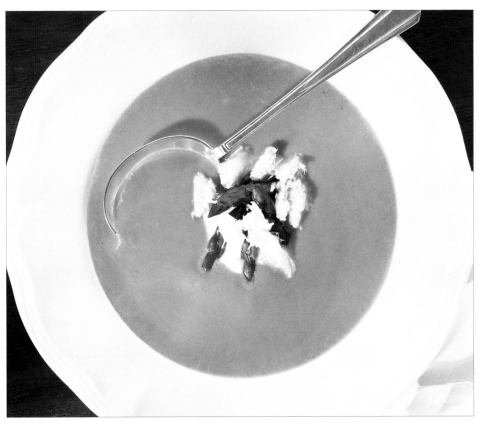

1 Trim the woody ends from the bottom of the asparagus spears and cut the spears into 2.5cm/1in pieces. Use scissors if it is easier.

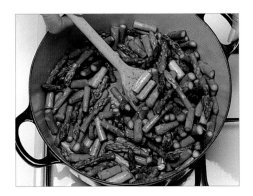

2 Heat the oil in a casserole or saucepan over a medium-high heat. Add the asparagus and cook for 5–6 minutes, stirring frequently, until bright green, but not browned.

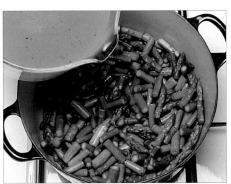

3 Add the stock and bring to the boil over a high heat, skimming off any foam that rises to the surface. Simmer over a medium heat for 3–5 minutes until the asparagus is tender, yet crisp. Reserve 12–16 of the asparagus tips for garnishing. Season with salt and pepper, cover and continue cooking for 15–20 minutes until very tender.

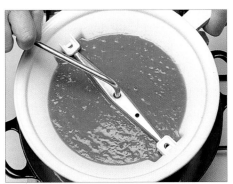

4 Purée the soup in a blender or food processor, or use a hand-held liquidizer. Pour the soup back into the saucepan. Bring it back to the boil over a medium-high heat.

5 Blend the cornflour with about 45ml/3 tbsp cold water and mix into the soup. Cook until thickened, then stir in the cream, if using. Season with salt and black pepper.

6 To serve, ladle the soup into bowls and top each with a spoonful of the crab meat and a few of the reserved asparagus tips.

NUTRITION NOTES

Per portion:

Energy	165kcals/676kJ
Fat, total	7.2g
saturated fat	1.9g
Protein	13.4g
Carbohydrate	12.1g
sugar, total	4.5g
Fibre – NSP	3.7g
Sodium	583mg

COOK'S TIP

If you have difficulty lifting, use a hand-held blender in the pan. The soup will be chunkier, but will still taste as good.

Green Lentil Soup

This is hearty North African soup is rich in the mineral selenium, an important antioxidant.

INGREDIENTS

Serves 4
225g/8oz/1 cup green lentils
75ml/5 tbsp olive oil
3 onions, finely chopped, or 45ml/
   3 tbsp dried onion
2 garlic cloves, thinly sliced, or 10ml/
   2 tsp garlic purée
10ml/2 tsp cumin seeds, crushed
1.5ml/¼ tsp ground turmeric
600ml/1 pint/2½ cups vegetable stock
salt and ground black pepper
30ml/2 tbsp roughly chopped fresh
   coriander, to serve
warm bread, to serve

1 Put the lentils in a pan and cover with cold water. Bring to the boil and boil rapidly for 10 minutes; drain.

2 Heat 30ml/2 tbsp of the oil in a deep saucepan and fry two of the onions (or 30ml/2 tbsp dried onion) with the garlic, cumin and turmeric for 3 minutes, stirring constantly.

3 Add the lentils and vegetable stock. Bring to the boil, then reduce the heat, cover and simmer gently for 30 minutes, until the lentils are soft.

4 Fry the third onion (or remaining 15ml/1 tbsp dried onion) in the remaining oil until golden.

5 Use a potato masher to lightly mash the lentils and make the soup pulpy. Reheat gently and season with salt and ground black pepper to taste. Pour the soup into serving bowls. Stir the chopped fresh coriander into the fried onion and scatter over the soup to decorate. Serve immediately, with warm bread.

COOK'S TIPS

• If you have difficulty lifting heavy pans, remove the lentils from their boiling water into the soup pot with a slotted spoon or ladle. If the lentils are really well cooked they will scarcely need mashing.
• If you prefer to use fresh onion and garlic, you can use an onion chopper to save you slicing them.

NUTRITION NOTES

Per portion:
Energy	320kcals/1312kJ
Fat, total	15.0g
saturated fat	2.0g
Protein	15.7g
Carbohydrate	32.6g
sugar, total	4.0g
Fibre – NSP	5.8g
Sodium	369mg

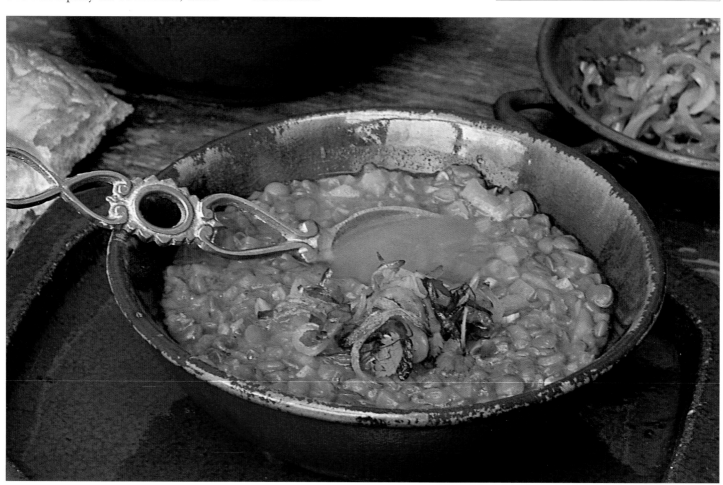

Spanish Garlic Soup

Topped with toasted French bread, this delicious and satisfying soup is almost a meal in itself. Try serving it for a winter lunch and let its wonderful aroma bring you a little Mediterranean sunshine.

INGREDIENTS

Serves 4

30ml/2 tbsp olive oil
4 large garlic cloves, peeled
4 slices French bread, 5mm/¼in thick, or if you are on a wheat-free diet, leave the bread out and have the soup just with the egg
15ml/1 tbsp paprika or, if you are on a solanacae-free diet, ground ginger
1 litre/1¾ pints/4 cups vegetable stock
1.5ml/¼ tsp ground cumin
pinch of saffron strands
4 eggs
salt and ground black pepper
chopped fresh parsley, to garnish

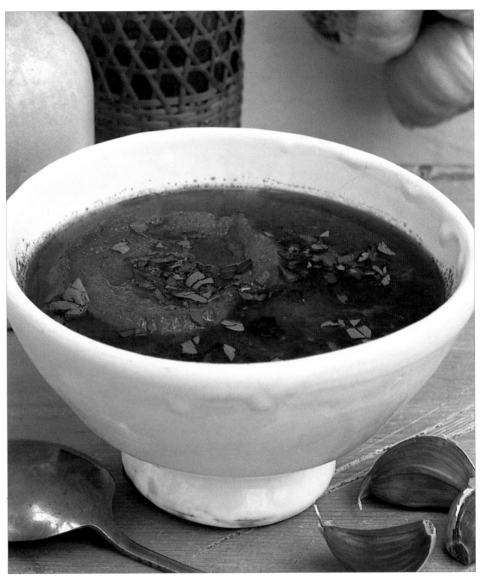

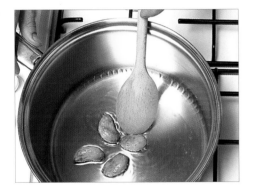

1 Preheat the oven to 230°C/450°F/ Gas 8. Heat the oil gently in a large pan. Add the whole garlic cloves and cook until golden. Remove and set aside. Toast the bread in the oven until it is golden.

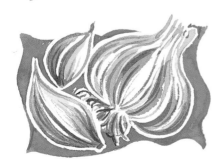

2 Add the paprika or ground ginger to the pan, and fry for a few seconds. Stir in the stock, cumin and saffron. Crush the reserved garlic cloves and add to the pan. Season with salt and pepper, and cook for about 5 minutes.

3 Ladle into four ovenproof bowls and break an egg into each. Place a slice of bread on each egg and bake in the oven for 3–4 minutes, until the eggs are set. Garnish with parsley; serve.

--- COOK'S TIPS ---

• To prevent the oil from overheating, add a tablespoon of water when frying the garlic.
• If you would find it difficult to put the soup bowls into the oven, you can either omit the eggs and serve the soup just with the bread and garlic, or poach the eggs all together in the soup and merely ladle them out with the soup.

--- NUTRITION NOTES ---

Per portion:

Energy	249kcals/1020kJ
Fat, total	12.8g
saturated fat	2.7g
Protein	12.3g
Carbohydrate	22.5g
sugar, total	0.8g
Fibre – NSP	0.6g
Sodium	668mg

Sorrel, Spinach and Salmon Soup

This is an excellent cold, Russian summer soup. It is traditionally made with *kvas*, a beer made from wheat, rye and buckwheat, but cider works equally well.

INGREDIENTS

Serves 4

30ml/2 tbsp olive oil
225g/8oz sorrel, washed and
  stalks removed
225g/8oz young spinach, washed and
  stalks removed
25g/1oz fresh horseradish, grated or
  15ml/1 tbsp grated horseradish in a jar
750ml/1¼ pints/3 cups cider
1 pickled cucumber, finely chopped
  or grated
30ml/2 tbsp chopped fresh dill, plus
  extra sprigs to garnish
225g/8oz cooked salmon, skinned
  and boned
salt and ground black pepper

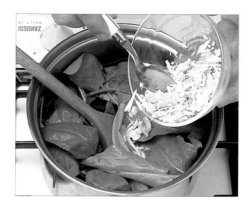

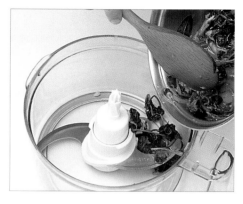

1 Heat the oil in a large pan. Add the sorrel and spinach leaves and the horseradish. Cover and cook gently for 3–4 minutes, or until the sorrel and spinach leaves are wilted.

2 Spoon the cooked leaves into a food processor and process to a fine purée, or purée with a hand-held processor. Ladle into a tureen or bowl and stir in the cider, pickled cucumber and chopped dill.

3 Chop the salmon into even, bite-size pieces. Add them to the soup, then season with plenty of salt and pepper to taste. Chill the soup for at least 3 hours before serving, garnished with a sprig of dill.

COOK'S TIP

If sorrel is unavailable, use double the amount of spinach instead and, just before serving, add a dash of lemon juice to the soup. Use vinegar if you are on a citrus-free diet.

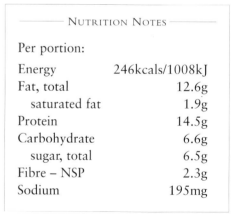

NUTRITION NOTES

Per portion:

Energy	246kcals/1008kJ
Fat, total	12.6g
saturated fat	1.9g
Protein	14.5g
Carbohydrate	6.6g
sugar, total	6.5g
Fibre – NSP	2.3g
Sodium	195mg

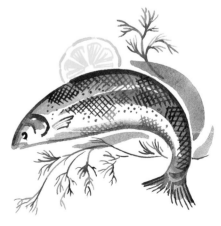

Carrot and Coriander Soup

Carrot and coriander are often combined in soups as their flavours are so complementary. This version uses soya milk, making it particularly suitable for people on a dairy-free diet.

INGREDIENTS

Serves 4

450g/1lb carrots, preferably young and tender
45ml/3 tbsp sunflower oil
1 onion, chopped or 30ml/2 tbsp dried onion
1 celery stick, sliced plus 2–3 pale leafy celery tops
2 small potatoes or, if you are on a solanacae-free diet, 1 sweet potato, peeled and cubed
1 litre/1¾ pints/4 cups chicken stock
10–15ml/2–3 tsp ground coriander
15ml/1 tbsp chopped fresh coriander
200ml/7fl oz/scant 1 cup soya milk
salt and ground black pepper

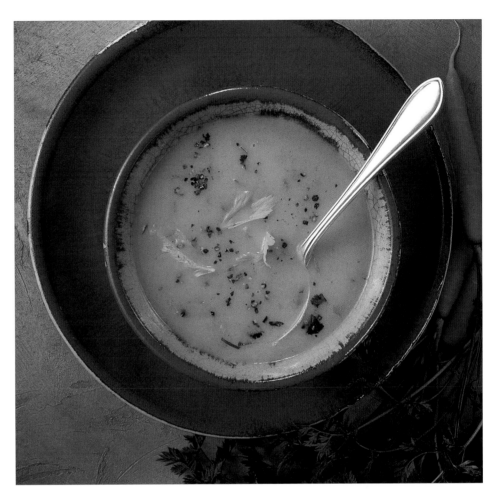

1 Trim the carrots, peel if necessary and cut into chunks. Heat 30ml/2 tbsp of the sunflower oil in a large pan and cook the onion over a gentle heat for 3–4 minutes until softened.

2 Add the sliced celery and potatoes or sweet potato to the onion in the saucepan, cook for a few minutes and then add the carrots. Fry the vegetables over a gentle heat for 3–4 minutes, stirring frequently, and then cover. Reduce the heat even further and sweat for about 10 minutes. Stir occasionally so the vegetables do not stick to the base of the pan.

3 Add the stock, bring to the boil and then partially cover and simmer for a further 8–10 minutes until the carrots and potatoes are tender.

4 Remove 6–8 tiny celery leaves for garnish and finely chop the remaining leaves (about 15ml/1 tbsp once chopped). Heat the remaining oil in a pan and fry the ground coriander for about 1 minute, stirring constantly.

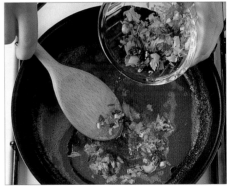

5 Reduce the heat and add the fresh coriander and celery leaves. Fry for about 1 minute. Set aside.

6 Process the soup in a food processor or blender or with a hand-held blender and pour back into the saucepan. Stir in the soya milk, coriander mixture and seasoning. Heat gently, taste and adjust the seasoning. Serve garnished with the reserved celery leaves.

COOK'S TIP

If you have difficulty with your hands you can leave the carrots, potato and celery whole and unpeeled – just make sure you wash them well. They will be much easier to cut up when cooked and soft. Alternatively, you could use dried vegetables.

NUTRITION NOTES

Per portion:

Energy	182kcals/746kJ
Fat, total	9.8g
saturated fat	1.3g
Protein	5.1g
Carbohydrate	19.3g
sugar, total	11.1g
Fibre – NSP	3.8g
Sodium	515mg

Dolmades

This tasty Greek dish of stuffed vine leaves has become a classic.

INGREDIENTS

Makes 24

28 fresh young vine leaves, soaked, or leaves from a packet or can
30ml/2 tbsp olive oil
1 large onion, finely chopped, or 30ml/2 tbsp dried onion
5ml/1 tsp garlic purée
225g/8oz/2 cups cooked long grain rice, or mixed white and wild rice
about 45ml/3 tbsp pine nuts
15ml/1 tbsp flaked almonds
40g/1½oz/¼ cup sultanas
15ml/1 tbsp snipped fresh chives
15ml/1 tbsp finely chopped fresh mint
juice of ½ lemon or, if you are on a citrus-free diet, 15ml/1 tbsp white wine vinegar
150ml/¼ pint/⅔ cup white wine
hot vegetable stock
salt and ground black pepper
fresh mint sprig, to garnish
natural yogurt and pitta bread, to serve (omit if you are on a dairy- or wheat-free diet)

1 If you are using fresh vine leaves, bring a pan of water to the boil and cook the vine leaves for 2–3 minutes. They will darken after about 1 minute, and simmering for a further minute or so will ensure they are pliable.

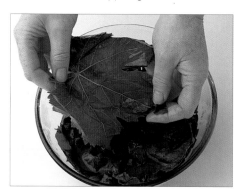

2 If using leaves from a packet or can, place them in a large bowl, cover with boiling water and leave for a few minutes until the leaves can easily be separated. Rinse them under cold water and drain on kitchen paper.

3 Heat the oil in a small frying pan and fry the onion and garlic gently for 3–4 minutes until soft. Spoon into a large bowl and add the cooked rice.

4 Stir in 30ml/2 tbsp of the pine nuts, the almonds, sultanas, chives and mint. Squeeze in the lemon juice or vinegar. Season to taste and mix well.

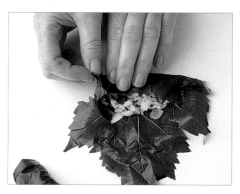

5 Set aside four large vine leaves. Lay a vine leaf on a clean work surface, veined side uppermost. Place a spoonful of filling near the stem, fold the lower part of the vine leaf over it and roll up, folding in the sides as you go. Stuff the rest in the same way.

6 Line the base of a deep frying pan or flameproof casserole dish with the reserved vine leaves. Place the dolmades close together in the pan, seam side down, in a single layer. Pour over the wine and enough stock to just cover. Anchor the dolmades by placing a plate on top of them, then cover the pan and simmer gently for 30 minutes.

7 Transfer the dolmades to a plate. Cool, chill, then garnish with the remaining pine nuts and the mint. Serve with a little yogurt and pitta bread, if you like.

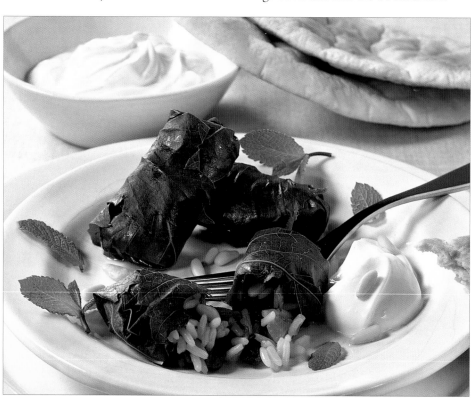

NUTRITION NOTES	
Per portion:	
Energy	69kcals/282kJ
Fat, total	2.9g
saturated fat	0.3g
Protein	1.4g
Carbohydrate	10.1g
sugar, total	1.8g
Fibre – NSP	0.3g
Sodium	70mg

Grilled Green Mussels with Cumin

Many people with osteoarthritis take green mussel supplements to help manage their condition – so this dish is not only delicious but excellent for your joints.

INGREDIENTS

Serves 4

45ml/3 tbsp fresh parsley
45ml/3 tbsp fresh coriander
1 garlic clove, crushed
pinch of ground cumin
25g/1oz/2 tbsp unsalted butter, or, if you are on a dairy-free diet, substitute 30ml/2 tbsp olive oil
25g/1oz/¼ cup brown breadcrumbs, or, if you are on a wheat-free diet, substitute 45ml/3 tbsp crushed plain potato crisps
ground black pepper
12 green mussels or 24 small mussels on the half-shell
fresh parsley leaves, to garnish

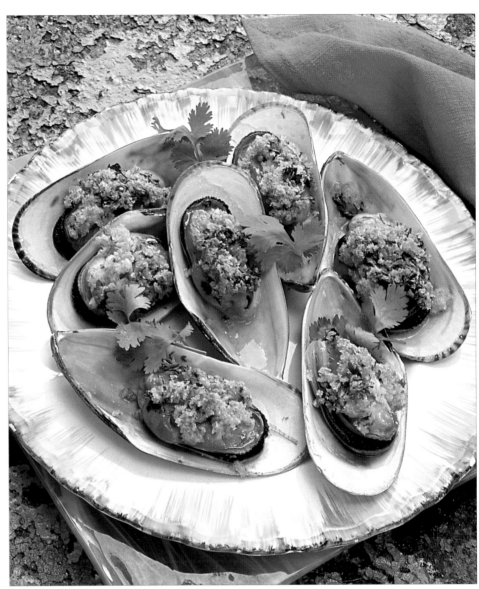

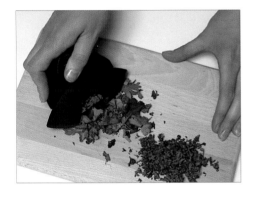

1 Chop the herbs finely. Use a broad-handled herb chopper or scissors if you find it easier.

NUTRITION NOTES

Per portion:

Energy	84kcals/344kJ
Fat, total	6.1g
saturated fat	3.8g
Protein	2.4g
Carbohydrate	5.3g
sugar, total	0.3g
Fibre – NSP	0.0g
Sodium	115mg

2 Beat the garlic, herbs, cumin and butter or oil together with a wooden spoon, or purée them together in a small food processor or coffee grinder.

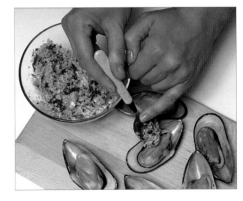

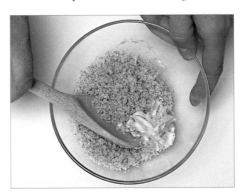

3 Stir in the breadcrumbs or crisps and the ground black pepper.

4 Carefully spoon a little of the mixture for the topping on to each mussel and cook under a medium-hot grill for 2 minutes. Serve the mussels immediately, garnished with the fresh parsley leaves.

Whiting Fillets with Polenta Crust

Whiting is a flaky, white fish with a delicate flavour, which the crisp polenta coating helps to seal in.

INGREDIENTS

Serves 4

8 small whiting fillets
finely grated rind of 1 lemon, or omit
    if on a citrus-free diet
225g/8oz/2 cups polenta
45ml/3 tbsp olive oil
salt and ground black pepper

To serve

30ml/2 tbsp chopped mixed fresh herbs
    such as parsley, chervil and chives,
    plus extra whole leaves
steamed spinach
red onion, sliced
toasted pine nuts

--- COOK'S TIPS ---

• Use quick-cooking polenta if you can, as it will give a better crunchy coating.
• If your hands are stiff, it may be easier to use scissors to chop the herbs.

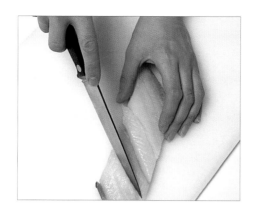

1 Make four small cuts in each fillet to stop the fish curling up when it is cooked.

--- NUTRITION NOTES ---

Per portion:

Energy	435kcals/1783kJ
Fat, total	10.6g
saturated fat	1.4g
Protein	40.6g
Carbohydrate	42.4g
sugar, total	0.0g
Fibre – NSP	0.0g
Sodium	191mg

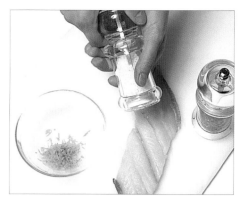

2 Season and, if using lemon rind, sprinkle most of it over the fish.

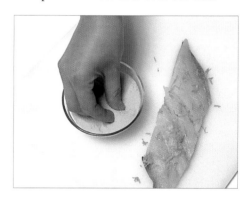

3 Press the polenta on to the fillets. Chill for 30 minutes.

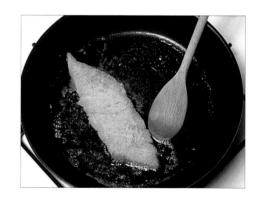

4 Heat the oil in a frying pan and fry for 3–4 minutes on each side. Garnish with the chopped herbs and herb leaves, and the reserved lemon rind. Serve with steamed spinach, sliced red onion and toasted pine nuts.

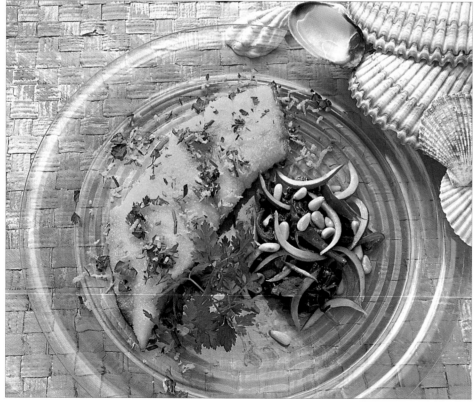

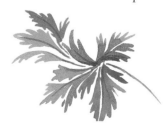

Sizzling Salmon with Herbs

Salmon is well known to arthritis sufferers for its anti-inflammatory properties. This is an unusual and exciting way to serve fresh salmon. A simple green salad makes a good side dish.

INGREDIENTS

Serves 4

4 salmon steaks, 175–200g/6–7oz each
30ml/2 tbsp olive oil
45ml/3 tbsp chopped fresh root ginger
   or 30ml/2 tbsp ground ginger
   or 45ml/3 tbsp ginger purée
90ml/6 tbsp chopped spring onions
90ml/6 tbsp chopped fresh coriander
50ml/2fl oz soy sauce, which should be
   wheat-free tamari if you are on a
   wheat-free diet, plus extra to serve
salt and ground black pepper
coriander sprigs, to garnish

1 Bring some water to a boil in the bottom of a steamer.

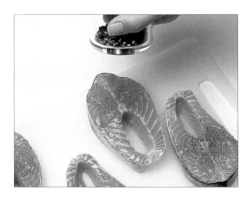

2 Season the fish steaks on both sides with salt and pepper.

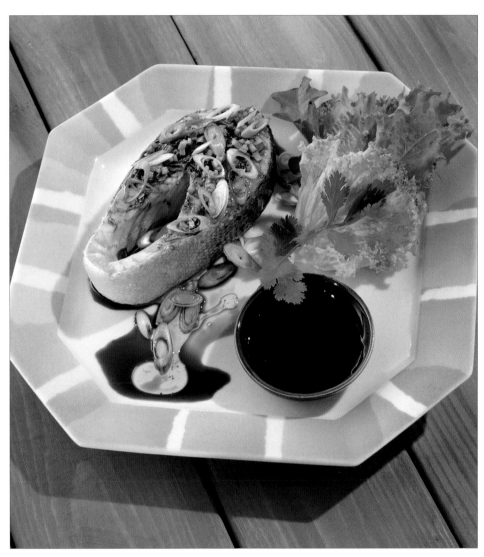

── NUTRITION NOTES ──	
Per portion:	
Energy	421kcals/1726kJ
Fat, total	27.5g
saturated fat	4.6g
Protein	41.9g
Carbohydrate	1.5g
sugar, total	0.3g
Fibre – NSP	0.1g
Sodium	948mg

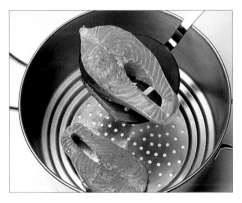

3 Place the fish steaks in the top part of the steamer. Cover the pan and steam the fish for 7–8 minutes, or until it is opaque all the way through.

4 Heat the oil and gently cook the root ginger, or ginger powder or purée, with the spring onions.

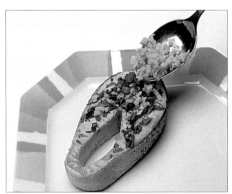

5 Place the salmon on warmed plates. Divide the chopped coriander among the salmon steaks. Spoon over the ginger and the spring onions. Drizzle 15ml/1 tbsp soy sauce over each salmon steak and serve with small bowls of extra soy sauce alongside. Garnish with coriander sprigs.

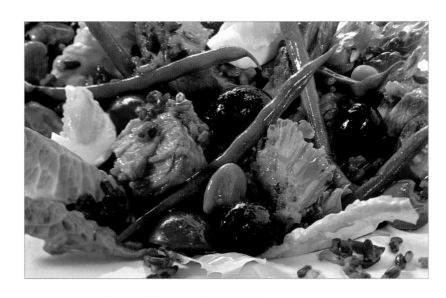

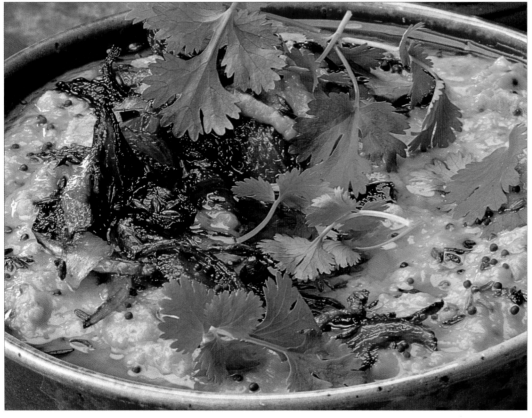

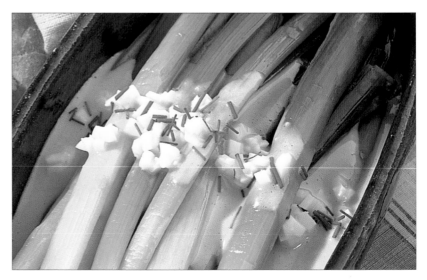

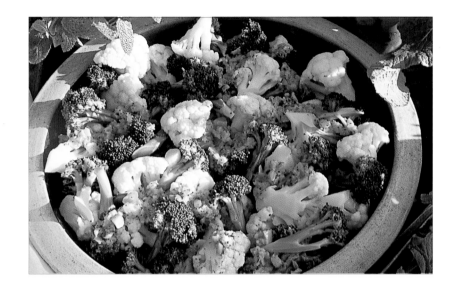

SALADS AND SIDE DISHES

A great selection of light dishes are included here, all of which are easy to

make and full of nutrients to help alleviate your arthritis.

Pasta salads are filling and tasty, and can include salmon or seeds to boost

your intake of inflammation-reducing GLAs and ALAs. Lentils are

a good choice when you are cutting down on meat consumption: try

the substantial Egyptian Rice with Lentils or the traditional Indian

Dhal with Tadka.

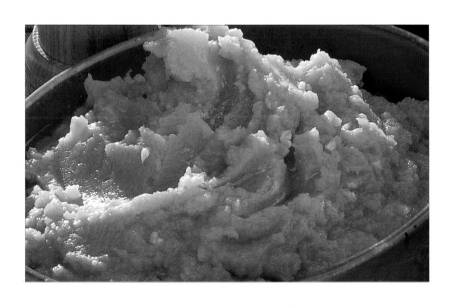

Smoked Salmon, Coconut and Dill Pasta

The coconut milk gives this dish an unusual and exotic flavour.

INGREDIENTS

Serves 4
350g/12oz/3 cups pasta twists, wheat-
    free if you are on a wheat-free diet
6 large sprigs fresh dill, chopped, plus
    more sprigs to garnish
30ml/2 tbsp extra virgin olive oil
15ml/1 tbsp white wine vinegar
300ml/½ pint/1¼ cups coconut cream
175g/6oz smoked salmon
salt and ground black pepper

1 Boil the pasta until just cooked.
Drain and rinse under the cold tap.

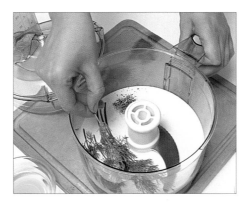

2 Make the dressing by combining all
the remaining ingredients, apart
from the smoked salmon and the dill
for the garnish, in the bowl of a food
processor. Alternatively, use a hand-
held blender in a bowl and blend well.

3 Slice the salmon into small strips
with scissors. Place the cooled pasta
and the smoked salmon in a serving
bowl. Pour on the dressing and toss
carefully. Garnish with the dill sprigs.

NUTRITION NOTES	
Per portion:	
Energy	678kcals/2779kJ
Fat, total	35.0g
saturated fat	23.8g
Protein	24.6g
Carbohydrate	70.5g
sugar, total	6.3g
Fibre – NSP	2.7g
Sodium	632mg

Avocado and Pasta Salad with Coriander

INGREDIENTS

Serves 4
900ml/1½ pints/3¾ cups chicken stock
225g/8oz/2 cups pasta bows, wheat-
    free if you are on a wheat-free diet
4 celery stalks, finely chopped
2 avocados, peeled and chopped
1 garlic clove, peeled and chopped, or
    2.5ml/½ tsp garlic purée
50g/2oz/½ cup mature Cheddar
    cheese, grated, or omit if you are on
    a dairy-free diet
15ml/1 tbsp chopped fresh coriander,
    plus some whole leaves to garnish
30ml/2 tbsp toasted sunflower seeds

For the dressing
150ml/¼ pint/⅔ cup extra virgin olive
    oil (cold pressed is best)
15ml/1 tbsp cider vinegar
30ml/2 tbsp lemon juice and grated
    rind of 1 lemon, or if you are on a
    citrus-free diet, use 45ml/3 tbsp
    vinegar and omit the rind
5ml/1 tsp Dijon mustard
15ml/1 tbsp chopped fresh coriander
salt and ground black pepper

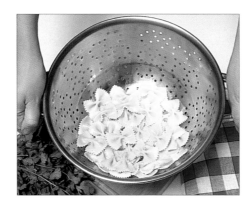

1 Bring the stock to the boil, add the
pasta, and simmer for 10 minutes
until cooked. Drain; set aside to cool.

NUTRITION NOTES	
Per portion:	
Energy	303kcals/1242kJ
Fat, total	13.9g
saturated fat	2.4g
Protein	10.2g
Carbohydrate	36.5g
sugar, total	1.6g
Fibre – NSP	3.7g
Sodium	643mg

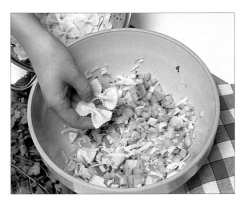

2 Mix the celery, avocados, garlic,
cheese and coriander in a bowl and
add the cooled pasta. Sprinkle with the
sunflower seeds.

3 To make the dressing, place all the
ingredients in a food processor or
coffee grinder and process until the
coriander is very finely chopped.
Alternatively, use a hand-held blender
in a bowl and blend well. Serve the
dressing separately, or pour over the
salad and toss before serving. Garnish
with coriander leaves.

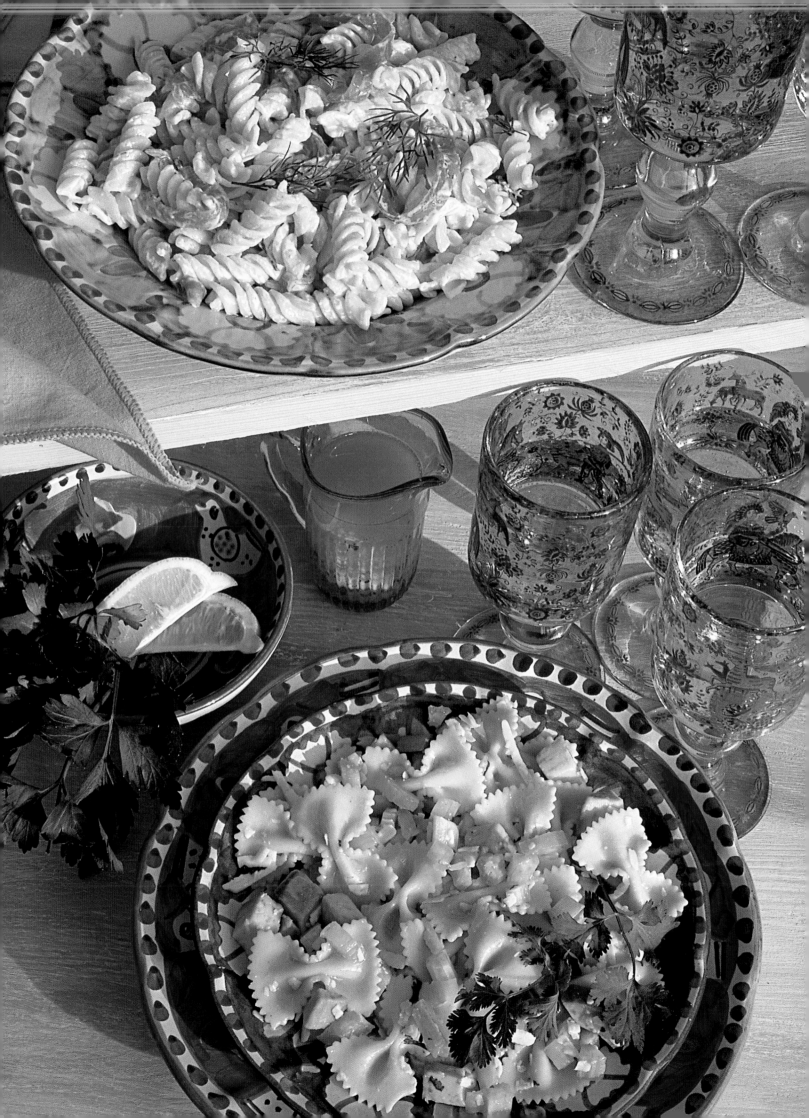

Red Rice Salad Niçoise

The sweet, nutty flavour of red rice makes a delicious variation on a classic Salad Niçoise. The thick steaks of fresh tuna make this tasty salad substantial enough to be a meal in its own right.

INGREDIENTS

Serves 6

about 675g/1½lb fresh tuna, sliced into 2cm/¾in thick steaks
350g/12oz/1¾ cups Camargue red rice
fish or vegetable stock or water
450g/1lb French beans
450g/1lb frozen and cooked, or drained, canned broad beans
1 cos lettuce
450g/1lb tiny cherry tomatoes or, if you are on a solanacae-free diet, omit and double the quantity of olives
30ml/2 tbsp fresh coriander, chopped
3 hard-boiled eggs (optional)
175g/6oz/1½ cups stoned black olives
olive oil, for brushing

For the marinade

1 onion, peeled and roughly chopped, or 30ml/2 tbsp dried onion
2 garlic cloves, peeled or 10ml/ 2 heaped tsp garlic purée
½ bunch fresh parsley
½ bunch fresh coriander
10ml/2 tsp paprika, or omit if you are on a solanacae-free diet
45ml/3 tbsp olive oil
45ml/3 tbsp water
30ml/2 tbsp white wine vinegar
15ml/1 tbsp fresh lime or lemon juice or, if you are on a citrus-free diet, 45ml/3 tbsp cider vinegar
salt and ground black pepper

For the dressing

30ml/2 tbsp fresh lime or lemon juice or, if you are on a citrus-free diet, cider vinegar
5ml/1 tsp Dijon mustard
½ garlic clove, crushed or 1.5ml/¼ tsp garlic purée (optional)
60ml/4 tbsp olive oil
60ml/4 tbsp sunflower oil

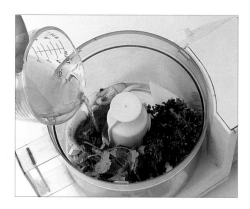

1 First, make the marinade for the tuna steaks. Place all the ingredients for the marinade in a food processor or blender and process for 30–40 seconds until all of the vegetables and herbs are finely chopped.

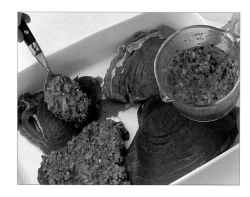

2 Prick the tuna steaks all over with a fork, then lay them side by side in a shallow dish. Spoon over the prepared marinade, turning the fish to coat each piece thoroughly.

3 Cover the dish with clear film and leave the tuna steaks to marinate in a cool place for 2–4 hours.

NUTRITION NOTES	
Per portion:	
Energy	638kcals/2615kJ
Fat, total	39.7g
saturated fat	27.1g
Protein	4.3g
Carbohydrate	58g
sugar, total	4.8g
Fibre – NSP	7.5g
Sodium	937mg

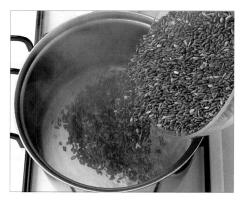

4 Cook the rice in the stock or water, following the instructions on the packet. Drain; set aside to cool.

5 To make the dressing, mix the citrus juice or cider vinegar, mustard and garlic, if using, in a bowl. Whisk in the oils, then add salt and pepper to taste. Stir 60ml/4 tbsp of the dressing into the rice, then spoon the rice into a large serving dish.

6 Steam the French beans until tender. Mix the French and broad beans into the rice. Discard the outer leaves from the lettuce and tear the inner ones into pieces. Add to the salad with the tomatoes, if using, and coriander. Shell the hard-boiled eggs, if using, and cut them into sixths. Preheat the grill.

7 Arrange the tuna steaks on the grill pan. Brush with the marinade and a little olive oil. Grill for 3–4 minutes on each side, until the fish is tender and flakes easily when tested with the tip of a sharp knife. Brush with marinade and more oil when turning the fish over.

8 Allow the fish to cool a little, then break it into large pieces. Toss into the salad with the olives and the remaining dressing. Decorate the salad with the eggs, if using, and serve.

VARIATION
This dish works well with swordfish steaks if tuna fish steaks aren't readily available.

Baked Fennel with a Crumb Crust

The delicate aniseed flavour of baked fennel goes well with tomatoes. Serve it with ratatouille or, if you are on a solanacae-free diet, with risotto. Fennel contains betacarotene, which the body converts into vitamin A.

INGREDIENTS

Serves 4

3 fennel bulbs, cut lengthways
   into quarters
30ml/2 tbsp olive oil
1 garlic clove, chopped or 5ml/1 tsp
   garlic purée
50g/2oz/½ cup day-old wholemeal
   breadcrumbs or, if you are on a
   wheat-free diet, 2 small packets of
   plain potato crisps, crushed
30ml/2 tbsp chopped fresh flat
   leaf parsley
salt and ground black pepper
fennel fronds, to garnish (optional)

COOK'S TIP

If you have difficulty using your hands, cook the fennel whole in the boiling water, remove with a slotted spoon and quarter when cooked, as it will be easier to cut.

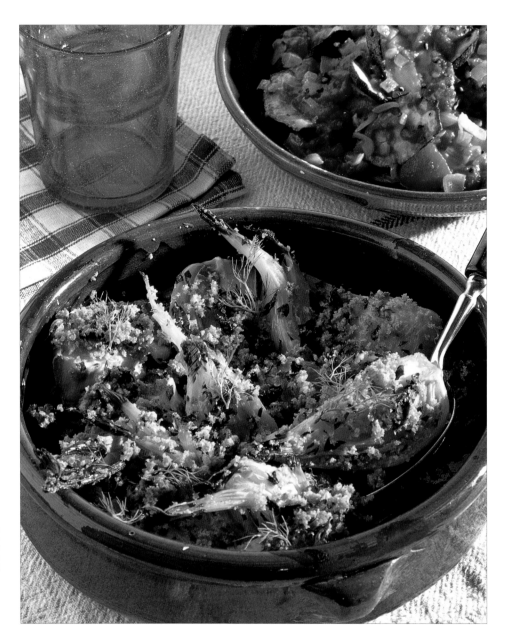

1 Cook the fennel in a saucepan of boiling salted water for 10 minutes or until just tender.

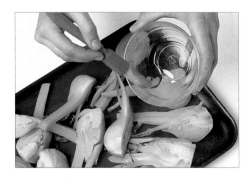

2 Drain the fennel and place them in a baking dish or roasting tin, then brush lightly with half of the olive oil. Meanwhile, preheat the oven to 190°C/375°F/Gas 5.

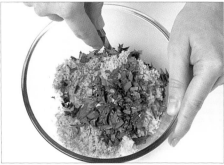

3 In a large mixing bowl, stir the garlic, breadcrumbs or crushed crisps and parsley together with the rest of the olive oil. Sprinkle the topping evenly over the fennel, then season well with salt and pepper.

4 Bake for 30 minutes until the crust is crisp and the fennel tender. Serve hot, garnished with a few fennel fronds.

NUTRITION NOTES

Per portion:

Energy	120kcals/492kJ
Fat, total	6.1g
saturated fat	0.8g
Protein	3.4g
Carbohydrate	13.7g
sugar, total	9.5g
Fibre – NSP	5.6g
Sodium	119mg

Carter's Millet

This dish was originally cooked over an open fire by carters who travelled across the steppes of southern Ukraine. It is a lovely filling dish for a chilly day.

INGREDIENTS

Serves 4

225g/8oz/scant 1¼ cups millet
600ml/1 pint/2½ cups vegetable stock
115g/4oz lardons or smoked streaky bacon with the rind removed, chopped
15ml/1 tbsp olive oil
1 small onion, chopped or 7.5ml/ 1½ tsp dried onion
225g/8oz/3 cups sliced or chopped small field mushrooms
15ml/1 tbsp chopped fresh mint
salt and ground black pepper

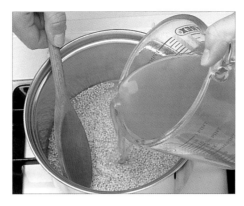

1 Rinse the millet in a sieve under cold running water. Put in a pan with the stock, bring to the boil and simmer, covered, for 30 minutes, until the stock has been absorbed.

2 Dry-fry the bacon in a non-stick pan for 5 minutes, or until brown and crisp. Remove and set aside.

3 Add the oil to the pan and cook the onion and mushrooms for 10 minutes, until starting to brown.

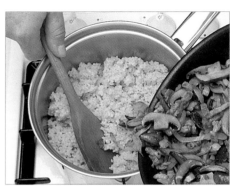

4 Add the cooked bacon, onion and mushrooms to the millet. Stir in the mint and season with salt and pepper. Heat gently for 1–2 minutes before serving.

COOK'S TIPS

The millet could be cooked in a table-top cooker or electric frying pan and the other ingredients added as they are ready. The dish can then be served from the pan. If fresh mint is not readily available, use flat leaf parsley or fresh coriander. Chop the bacon with scissors if you find this easier.

NUTRITION NOTES

Per portion:

Energy	332kcals/1361kJ
Fat, total	10.9g
saturated fat	2.8g
Protein	10.6g
Carbohydrate	46.0g
sugar, total	0.5g
Fibre – NSP	1.1g
Sodium	738mg

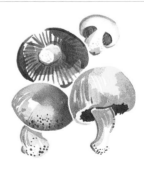

Egyptian Rice with Lentils

This is a simple, highly nutritious and very filling dish. It can be served as a main course accompaniment or simply enjoyed as a meal in itself.

INGREDIENTS

Serves 6

350g/12oz/1½ cups large brown lentils, soaked overnight in water
2 large onions or 60ml/4 tbsp dried onion
45ml/3 tbsp olive oil
15ml/1 tbsp ground cumin
2.5ml/½ tsp ground cinnamon
225g/8oz/generous 1 cup long grain rice
salt and ground black pepper
flat leaf parsley, to garnish

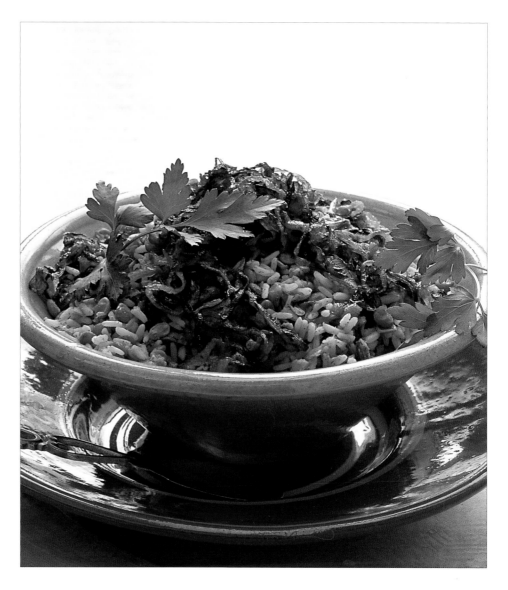

1 Drain the lentils and put them in the top of a steamer. Put enough water in the bottom of the steamer to cover the lentils by 5cm/2in.

2 Bring the water to the boil, cover the pan and simmer for 40 minutes to 1½ hours, or until the lentils are tender. Remove the top of the steamer with the lentils and drain.

3 Slice one of the onions very finely. Chop the other onion. Heat 15ml/1 tbsp of the olive oil in a saucepan, add the chopped onion and fry until soft.

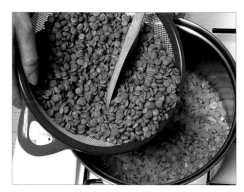

4 Add the drained lentils to the pan. Season with salt and pepper, then add the cumin and cinnamon.

5 Measure the volume of rice and add it, with the same volume of water, to the lentil mixture. Cover the saucepan and simmer for about 20 minutes, or until the rice is tender.

6 Heat the remaining olive oil in a frying pan, and cook the sliced onion until very dark brown.

COOK'S TIPS

• If you would find it difficult to slice the onion for the topping, chop both onions as finely as you can.
• Cook the chopped onion in a table-top cooker, then add the lentils and rice. The dish can then be served from the cooker.

7 Tip the rice and lentil mixture into a serving bowl and sprinkle the fried onion over the top. Garnish with flat leaf parsley. This dish can be served hot or cold.

NUTRITION NOTES

Per portion:

Energy	380kcals/1558kJ
Fat, total	8.0g
saturated fat	1.2g
Protein	17.4g
Carbohydrate	63.8g
sugar, total	2.9g
Fibre – NSP	5.9g
Sodium	9.7mg

Dhal with Tadka

Serve this aromatic Indian dish with naan bread or a wheat-free bread, if you like, to mop up the delicious sauce.

INGREDIENTS

Serves 4

45ml/3 tbsp olive or sunflower oil
10ml/2 tsp black mustard seeds
1 onion, finely chopped or 10ml/2 tsp dried onion
2 garlic cloves, finely chopped or 10ml/2 tsp garlic purée
5ml/1 tsp ground turmeric
5ml/1 tsp ground cumin
2 fresh green chillies, seeded and finely chopped or, if you are on a solanacae-free diet, 50g/2oz piece of ginger, peeled and finely chopped, or 10ml/2 tsp powdered ginger
225g/8oz/1 cup red lentils
300ml/½ pint/1¼ cups canned coconut milk
1 quantity tadka (see Cook's Tip)
fresh coriander sprigs, to garnish

---

1 Heat the oil in a large saucepan or frying pan. Add the mustard seeds. When they start to pop, add the onion and garlic and cook for 5–10 minutes until soft.

VARIATION

This dish is also excellent made with yellow split peas. Like lentils, split peas do not hold their shape when cooked, making them perfect for dhals.

NUTRITION NOTES

Per portion:

Energy	258kcals/1057kJ
Fat, total	6.5g
saturated fat	1.0g
Protein	14.0g
Carbohydrate	38.3g
sugar, total	7.1g
Fibre – NSP	3.3g
Sodium	103.8mg

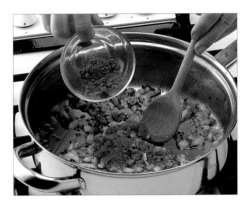

2 Stir in the turmeric, cumin and chillies or ginger and cook for 2 minutes. Add the lentils with 1 litre/1¾ pints/4 cups water and the coconut milk and bring to the boil.

3 Cover the saucepan and simmer for about 40 minutes, adding water if necessary. The lentils should be soft and should have absorbed most of the liquid. Transfer the dhal to a serving dish and keep warm.

4 Follow the instructions in the Cook's Tip to prepare the tadka, then pour over the dhal. Garnish with coriander sprigs and serve immediately.

COOK'S TIP

A tadka is a mixture of spices and flavourings fried in mustard oil to release their flavours, then added to Indian dishes such as dhal or vegetables.

INGREDIENTS

60ml/4 tbsp mustard oil
45-60ml/3–4 tbsp cumin seeds
1 small onion, finely chopped
60ml/4 tbsp finely chopped fresh coriander

1 Heat the mustard oil until it is just smoking, then turn off the heat and allow the oil to cool briefly.
2 Reheat the oil and fry the cumin seeds until they change colour. Add the onion and cook until it turns golden.
3 Finally, add the coriander and stir for a few seconds, then pour the mixture over the dhal.

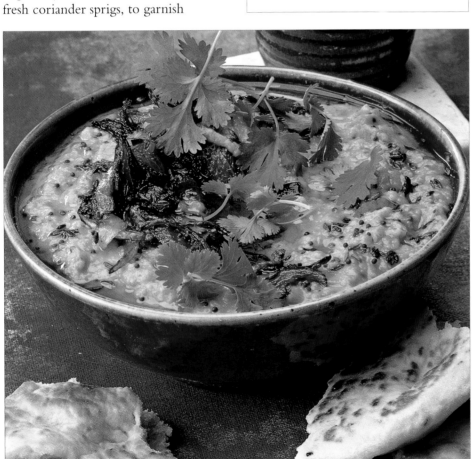

Garlic Sweet Potato Mash

Orange-fleshed sweet potatoes are delicious mashed with garlic-flavoured olive or walnut oil. Sweet potatoes are packed with vitamins too. They are not members of the potato family, so they are ideal if you are on a solanacae-free diet.

INGREDIENTS

Serves 4

4 large sweet potatoes, peeled, total weight about 900g/2lb, cubed
45ml/3 tbsp walnut or olive oil
3 garlic cloves, crushed or 10ml/2 tsp garlic purée
salt and ground black pepper

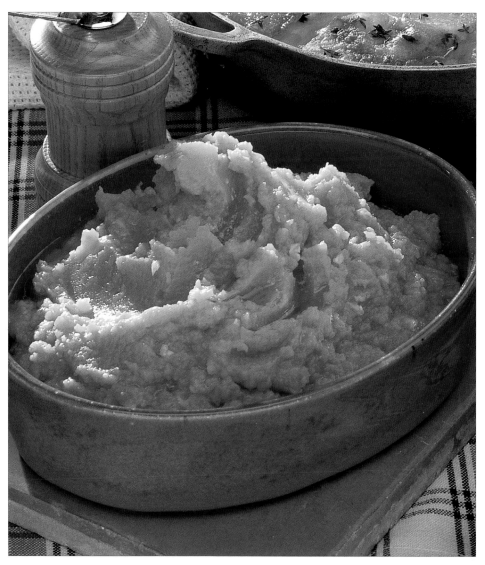

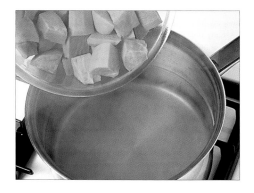

1 Place the sweet potatoes in a saucepan containing boiling water and cook for about 15 minutes or until tender. Cook them in the top half of a steamer if that is easier.

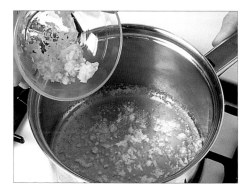

2 Heat the oil in a saucepan, then sauté the garlic over a low to medium heat for 1–2 minutes until light golden, stirring to prevent the garlic burning.

3 Pour the garlic oil over the sweet potatoes and season with salt and plenty of black pepper. Mash thoroughly until smooth and creamy. Serve immediately while the potatoes are piping hot.

NUTRITION NOTES	
Per portion:	
Energy	269kcals/1102kJ
Fat, total	8.9g
saturated fat	1.4g
Protein	2.7g
Carbohydrate	47.9g
sugar, total	12.8g
Fibre – NSP	5.4g
Sodium	90.0mg

COOK'S TIPS

• Sweet potatoes have quite tough skins so they do need to be peeled. If you find this difficult, cook them first and peel them once cooked – it is easier.
• If the potatoes seem rather dry when you are mashing them, add a little milk.
• If you have difficulty mashing by hand you can use a hand-held blender.

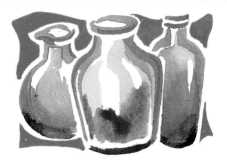

Warm Leeks with Vinaigrette

Use tender baby leeks for this dish if you can find them, and unless you are on a wheat-free diet, mop up the vinaigrette with thick chunks of crusty bread.

INGREDIENTS

Serves 6

12 small leeks (total weight about
   1.3kg/3lb)
2 eggs, hard-boiled
15ml/1 tbsp Dijon mustard
30ml/2 tbsp lemon juice or, if you are on
   a citrus-free diet, white wine vinegar
90ml/6 tbsp sunflower oil
90ml/6 tbsp extra virgin olive oil, plus
   more if needed
salt and ground black pepper
15–30ml/1–2 tbsp snipped fresh chives,
   to garnish

1 Remove the dark tough outer leaves of the leeks, then cut all the leeks to roughly the same length, and trim the dark green tops.

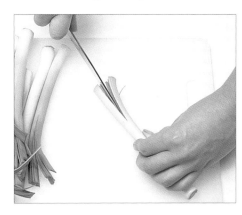

2 Trim the root ends, leaving enough to hold the leeks together, then split the top half of the leeks lengthways and rinse well under cold running water.

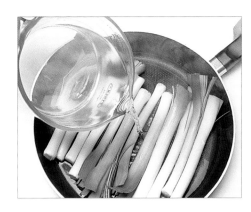

3 Lay the leeks flat in a large frying pan, pour over enough boiling water to just cover them and add a little salt. Cook the leeks over a medium-high heat for 7–10 minutes until just tender. Carefully remove the leeks with a slotted spoon, then lay them on a dish towel and press them gently to remove as much liquid as possible.

4 In a bowl, mash together the hard-boiled egg yolks and mustard to form a smooth paste. Season and add the lemon juice or vinegar, stirring until smooth. Slowly whisk in the sunflower oil, followed by the olive oil to make a thick, creamy vinaigrette. You can also whisk the vinaigrette together in a food processor, or in a bowl with a hand-held blender.

5 Arrange the leeks in a serving dish and pour over the vinaigrette while the leeks are still warm. Chop the egg whites and sprinkle them over the leeks, then scatter over the snipped fresh chives and serve warm or at room temperature.

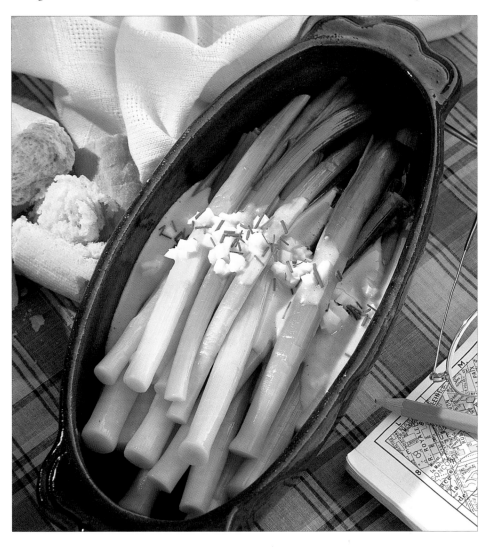

NUTRITION NOTES	
Per portion:	
Energy	272kcals/1115kJ
Fat, total	25.1g
saturated fat	3.6g
Protein	5.8g
Carbohydrate	6.2g
sugar, total	4.7g
Fibre – NSP	4.7g
Sodium	30.9mg

Braised Red Cabbage

This dish is a wonderful deep-red colour and has a rich and sweet flavour.

INGREDIENTS

Serves 8

30ml/2 tbsp olive oil

2 medium onions, thinly sliced or chopped or 45ml/3 tbsp dried onion

2 eating apples, peeled, cored and thinly sliced or, if peeling the apples is difficult, leave the skins on and chop them roughly

1 head red cabbage (about 900g–1.2kg/ 2–2½lb), trimmed, cored, halved and thinly sliced

60ml/4 tbsp red wine vinegar

15–30ml/1–2 tbsp sugar

1.5ml/¼ tsp ground cloves

5–10ml/1–2 tsp mustard seeds

50g/2oz/⅓ cup raisins or currants

about 120ml/4fl oz/½ cup red wine or water

15–30ml/1–2 tbsp redcurrant jelly (optional)

salt and ground black pepper

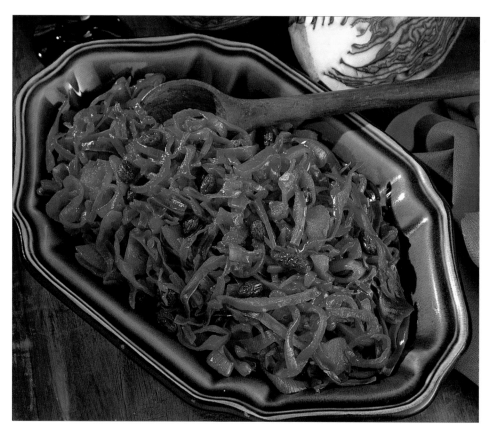

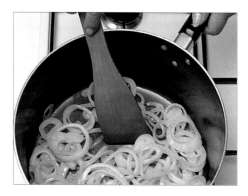

1 Heat the olive oil over a medium heat. Add the onions and cook for 7–10 minutes until they are golden.

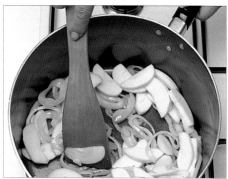

2 Add the apples to the pan and cook, stirring continuously, for 2–3 minutes until they are just softened.

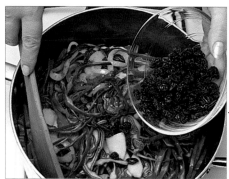

3 Add the cabbage, red wine vinegar, sugar, cloves, mustard seeds, raisins or currants, red wine or water and salt and pepper, stirring until well mixed. Bring to the boil over a medium-high heat, stirring occasionally.

4 Cover and cook over a medium-low heat for 35–40 minutes until the cabbage is tender and the liquid is just absorbed, stirring occasionally. Add a little more red wine or water if the pan boils dry before the cabbage is tender. Just before serving, stir in the redcurrant jelly, if using, to sweeten and glaze the cabbage.

COOK'S TIPS

• If you find the cabbage difficult to cut up, use a long or double knife so that you can lean on both ends, and cut it on an old dish towel to stop it slipping.

• The whole dish could be cooked in, and served from, a table-top cooker.

NUTRITION NOTES

Per portion:

Energy	101kcals/414kJ
Fat, total	3.1g
saturated fat	0.2g
Protein	1.8g
Carbohydrate	17.6g
sugar, total	16.7g
Fibre – NSP	3.8g
Sodium	15.6mg

Broccoli and Cauliflower with Cider

The sauce in this dish is a good way of enhancing lightly steamed vegetables. It can be served with rice as a simple vegetarian meal.

INGREDIENTS

Serves 4
30ml/2 tbsp olive oil
1 large onion, chopped or 30ml/2 tbsp dried onion
2 large carrots, chopped
1 large clove garlic or 2.5ml/½ tsp garlic purée
15ml/1 tbsp dill seed
4 large sprigs apple mint
30ml/2 tbsp plain flour or, if you are on a wheat-free diet, use potato or cornflour
300ml/½ pint/1¼ cups cider
30ml/2 tbsp soy sauce or, if you are on a wheat-free diet, wheat-free tamari
10ml/2 tsp mint jelly
450g/1lb broccoli florets
450g/1lb cauliflower florets

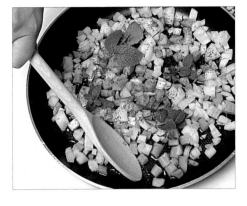

1 Heat the olive oil in a large saucepan or frying pan. Add the onion, carrots, garlic, dill seed and apple mint leaves and sauté over a medium heat until the vegetables are nearly cooked.

2 Meanwhile, steam the broccoli and cauliflower florets for 10 minutes or until just tender, then transfer to a large serving bowl. Keep the broccoli and cauliflower florets warm while you finish making the sauce.

3 Stir the flour into the sautéed vegetables. Then pour in the cider and simmer until the sauce looks glossy.

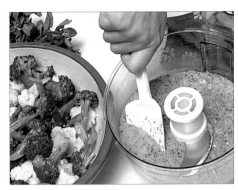

4 Pour the sautéed vegetables into a food processor. Add the soy sauce or tamari and the mint jelly and blend until finely puréed. If you like, return the sauce to the pan and heat through gently. Pour the warm sauce over the broccoli and cauliflower florets and serve immediaely.

COOK'S TIPS

• If you would have difficulty chopping the vegetables for the sauce, you can cook them whole instead. They will be much easier to chop once they are cooked.
• Tamari is a type of soy sauce that does not contain wheat.
• You may find it easier to liquidize the vegetables for the sauce in the saucepan, using a hand-held blender.
• Try adding sunflower or pumpkin seeds to this dish. They contain GLAs which have been shown to reduce inflammation.

NUTRITION NOTES

Per portion:

Energy	182kcals/746kJ
Fat, total	7.7g
saturated fat	1.3g
Protein	9.9g
Carbohydrate	13.8g
sugar, total	11.4g
Fibre – NSP	6.5g
Sodium	38.1mg

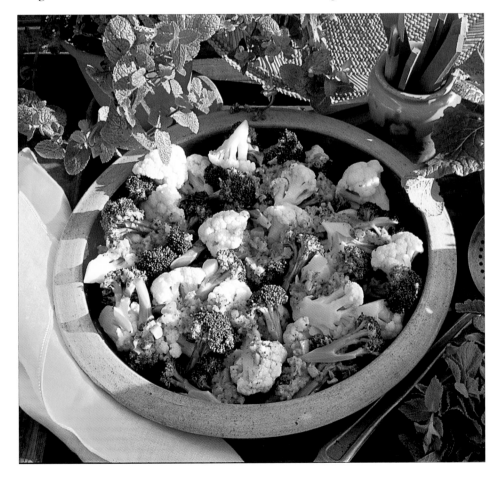

Soused Herrings

Herrings are an oily fish, full of the nutrients that have been shown to reduce inflammation.

INGREDIENTS

Serves 4
4 herrings
150ml/¼ pint/⅔ cup white wine vinegar
10ml/2 tsp salt
12 black peppercorns
2 bay leaves
4 whole cloves
2 small onions, sliced or 7.5ml/ 1 heaped tsp dried onion
bay leaves, to garnish

For the dressing
5ml/1 tsp coarse grain mustard
45ml/3 tbsp olive oil
15ml/1 tbsp white wine vinegar
salt and ground black pepper

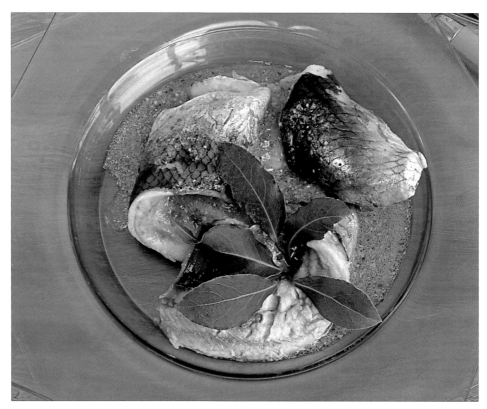

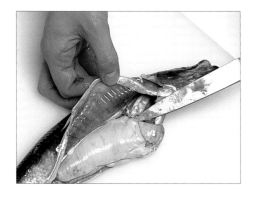

1 Preheat the oven to 160°C/325°F/ Gas 3. Clean and bone the fish, if necessary, and use a sharp knife to divide each fish into two fillets.

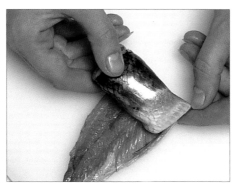

2 Roll up the fillets tightly and place them closely packed together in an ovenproof dish so that they can't unroll.

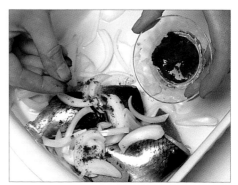

4 Add the salt, spices and onions and bake for 1 hour. Leave the herring to cool in the liquid. Meanwhile, make the dressing. Whisk all the ingredients with a fork in a small bowl, or place in a screw-top jar and shake until combined. Garnish the fish with bay leaves and serve with the dressing.

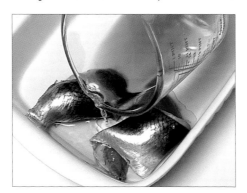

3 Pour the vinegar over the top and add water to just cover the fish.

— NUTRITION NOTES —

Per portion:

Energy	420kcals/1722kJ
Fat, total	31.4g
saturated fat	6.9g
Protein	31.6g
Carbohydrate	2.9g
sugar, total	2.1g
Fibre – NSP	0.5g
Sodium	211mg

— COOK'S TIPS —

• Buy the herring ready boned and cleaned to make this dish easier to prepare.
• The fish do not need to be rolled up but can be layered in a pan to cook if you find them difficult to handle.

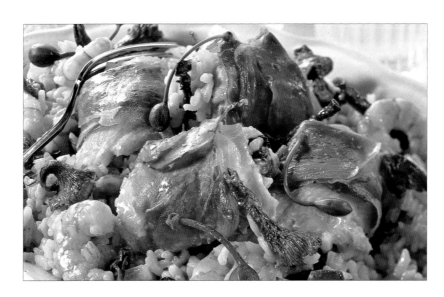

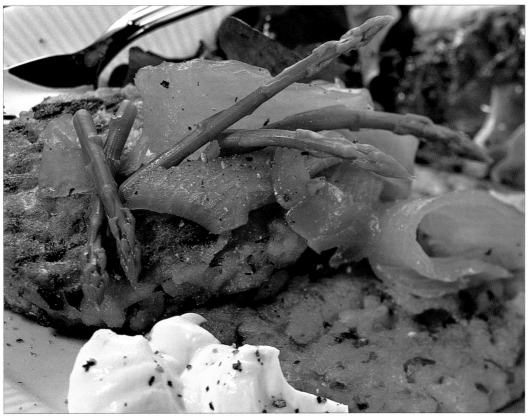

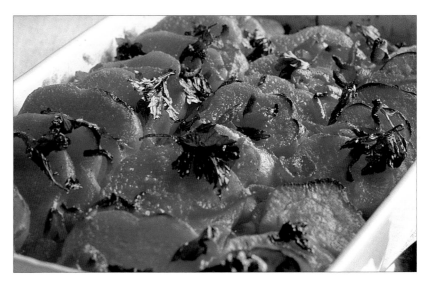

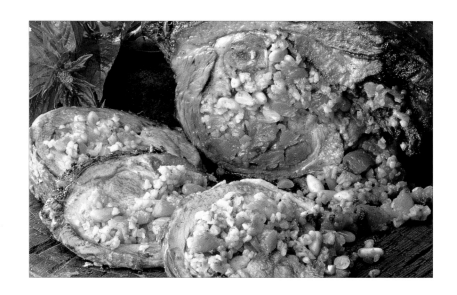

FISH AND MEAT DISHES

Oily fish such as salmon, mackerel and sardines contain beneficial

nutrients which can reduce inflammation in joints swollen by arthritis,

and you will find many recipes using oily fish in this section.

Or try a meat dish lower in fat such as Chicken with Mangetouts

and Ginger or Glazed Sweet Potatoes with Bacon. All of the recipes

can be adapted easily to avoid the common arthritis trigger foods for

those who are following a special diet.

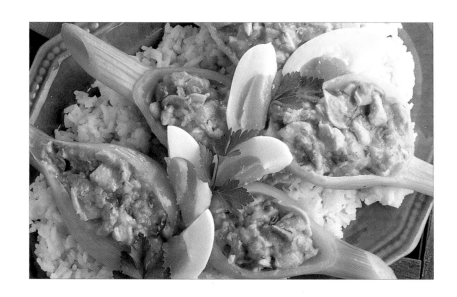

Salmon Steaks with Sorrel

Salmon and fresh leaves are traditionally paired in French cooking – the sharp flavour of the sorrel balances the richness of the fish. If sorrel is not available use chopped watercress instead.

INGREDIENTS

Serves 2

2 salmon steaks (about 250g/9oz each)
30ml/2 tbsp olive oil
2 shallots, finely chopped or 15ml/
 1 tbsp dried onion
45ml/3 tbsp whipping cream or, if you
 are on a dairy-free diet, soya cream
90g/3½oz fresh sorrel leaves, washed
 and patted dry
salt and ground black pepper
fresh sage, to garnish

1 Season the salmon steaks with salt and freshly ground black pepper to taste. In a large saucepan, heat half of the oil over a medium heat. Add the chopped shallots or dried onion and fry for 3–4 minutes, stirring frequently, until just softened.

NUTRITION NOTES	
Per portion:	
Energy	646kcals/2771kJ
Fat, total	47.7g
saturated fat	11.9g
Protein	52.4g
Carbohydrate	1.8g
sugar, total	1.8g
Fibre – NSP	1.1g
Sodium	185mg

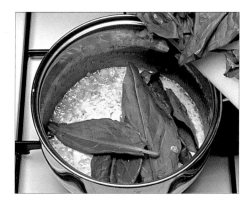

2 Add the cream and sorrel and cook for 3–4 minutes until the sorrel is completely wilted, stirring constantly.

3 Meanwhile, brush a non-stick frying pan with the remaining oil. Place over a medium heat until the olive oil is hot.

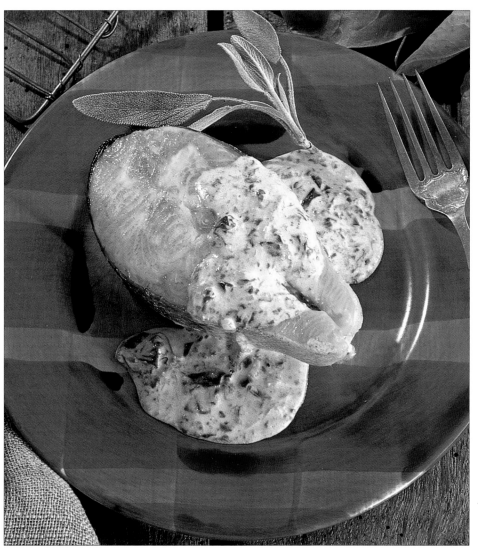

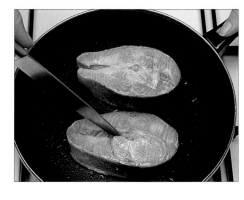

4 Add the salmon steaks to the frying pan and cook for about 5 minutes, turning once, until the flesh is opaque next to the bone. If you're not sure, pierce the salmon steaks with the tip of a sharp knife; if the fish are done the juices will run clear.

5 Arrange the salmon steaks on two warmed plates, garnish with sage and serve with the sorrel sauce.

COOK'S TIP
If your hands are weak you may find it easier to cook the salmon steaks in a microwave oven for 4–5 minutes, in a tightly covered container, or according to the manufacturer's guidelines.

Grilled Mackerel with Spicy Dhal

Oily fish such as mackerel and sardines are often complemented by a tart accompaniment. In this recipe they are served with tamarind-flavoured lentils.

INGREDIENTS

Serves 4

250g/9oz/1 cup red lentils, or yellow
   split peas (soaked overnight)
1 litre/1¾ pints/4 cups water
30ml/2 tbsp sunflower oil
2.5ml/½ tsp each mustard seeds, fennel
   seeds, cumin seeds and fenugreek seeds
5ml/1 tsp ground turmeric
3–4 dried red chillies, crumbled, or
   omit if you are on a solanacae-free diet
30ml/2 tbsp tamarind paste
5ml/1 tsp soft brown sugar
30ml/2 tbsp chopped fresh coriander
4 mackerel or 8 fresh sardines, cleaned
salt and ground black pepper
finely chopped coriander and fresh red
   chilli slices (optional), to garnish
chapatis, to serve (optional)

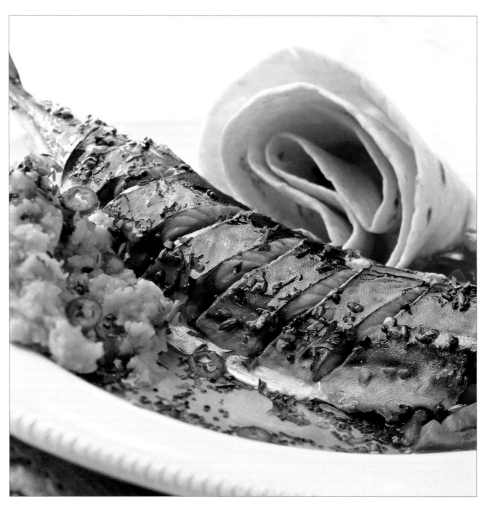

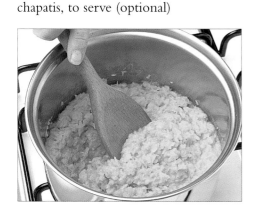

1 Rinse the lentils or split peas, drain and put them in a saucepan. Add the water and bring to the boil, then lower the heat, partially cover the pan and simmer for 30–40 minutes, stirring occasionally, until the pulses are tender.

—————— COOK'S TIP ——————

If you have problems lifting heavy pans, remove the pulses from their cooking water using a slotted spoon. Empty the pan when the water is cold, which is much safer.

2 Heat the oil and add the mustard seeds. Cover and cook for a few seconds, until they pop. Add the other seeds, with the turmeric and chillies, if using, and fry for a few more seconds.

3 Stir in the pulses and season. Mix well; stir in the tamarind paste and sugar. Bring to the boil, then simmer for 10 minutes. Stir in the coriander.

——————— NUTRITION NOTES ———————

Per portion:

Energy	688kcals/2820kJ
Fat, total	38.1g
saturated fat	7.3g
Protein	53.0g
Carbohydrate	35.1g
sugar, total	1.5g
Fibre – NSP	3.0g
Sodium	138.5mg

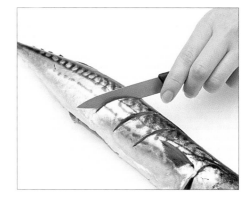

4 Heat the grill or a ridged grilling pan until very hot. Make six diagonal slashes on either side of each fish. Season inside and out.

5 Grill the fish for 5–7 minutes on each side, until the skin is blistered and crisp. Place each fish on a plate with the dhal and garnish with coriander and chillis, if using. If you like, serve with chapatis, wheat-free if necessary.

Trout and Parma Ham Risotto Rolls

This is an imaginative dinner party dish which is bound to impress.

Ingredients

Serves 4
4 trout fillets, skinned
Parma ham, 4 slices
caper berries, to garnish

For the risotto
30ml/2 tbsp olive oil
8 large raw prawns, peeled and deveined
1 onion, chopped
225g/8oz/generous 1 cup risotto rice
about 105ml/7 tbsp white wine
about 750ml/1¼ pints/3 cups
　simmering fish or chicken stock
15g/½oz/2 tbsp dried porcini or
　chanterelle mushrooms, soaked for
　10 minutes in warm water to cover
salt and ground black pepper

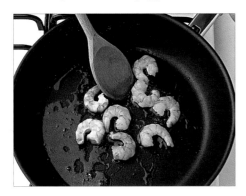

1 Heat the oil in a deep frying pan or table-top cooker and fry the prawns very briefly until flecked with pink. Lift out on a slotted spoon and transfer to a plate.

2 Add the chopped onion to the oil remaining in the pan and fry over a gentle heat for 3–4 minutes until soft.

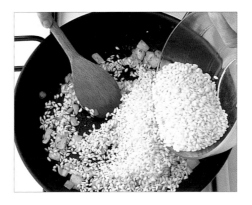

3 Add the rice to the pan and stir for 3–4 minutes until the grains are evenly coated in oil. Add 75ml/5 tbsp of the wine and then the stock, a little at a time, stirring over a gentle heat and allowing the rice to absorb the liquid before adding more.

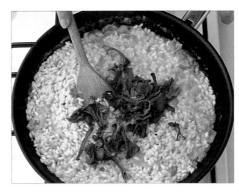

4 Drain the mushrooms, reserving the liquid, and cut the larger ones in half. Towards the end of cooking, stir the mushrooms into the risotto with 15ml/1 tbsp of the reserved mushroom liquid. Season to taste with salt and pepper.

─── Nutrition Notes ───

Per portion:

Energy	513kcals/2103kJ
Fat, total	15.8g
saturated fat	6.3g
Protein	41.5g
Carbohydrate	45.8g
sugar, total	2.3g
Fibre – NSP	7.3g
Sodium	842mg

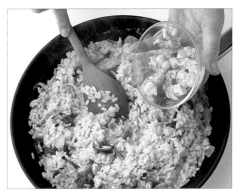

5 Remove the pan from the heat and stir in the prawns. Preheat the oven to 190°C/375°F/Gas 5.

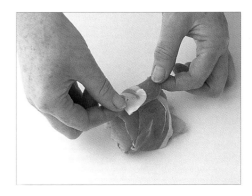

6 Take each trout fillet in turn, place a spoonful of risotto at one end and roll up. Wrap in a slice of Parma ham and place in a greased ovenproof dish.

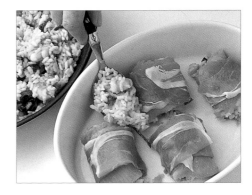

7 Spoon any remaining risotto around the fish fillets and sprinkle over the rest of the wine. Cover loosely with foil and bake for 15–20 minutes until the fish is tender. Spoon the risotto on to a platter, top with the trout rolls and garnish with capers. Unless you are on a wheat-free diet, wholemeal bread goes well with this.

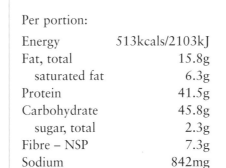

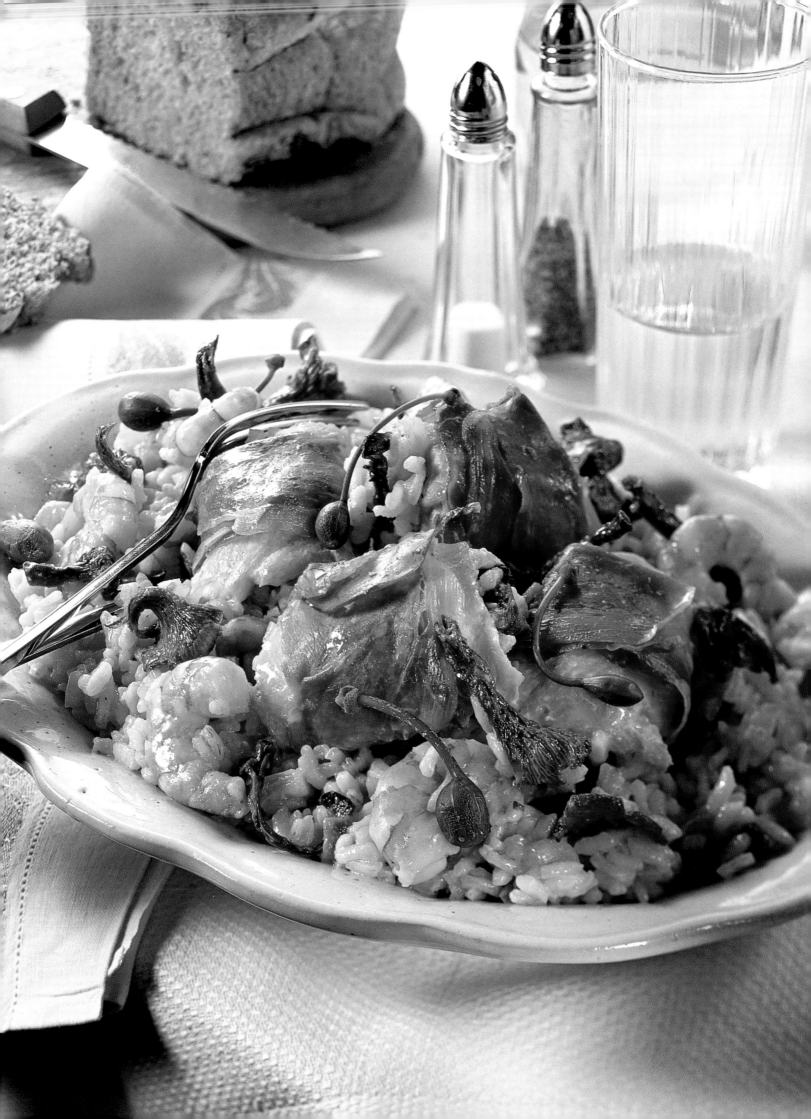

Tuscan Tuna and Beans

A classic Italian mixture – tasty, filling and healthy. It's quick to make if you're short of time.

INGREDIENTS

Serves 4

1 red onion, or 6 spring onions, trimmed
30ml/2 tbsp smooth French mustard
300ml/½ pint/1¼ cups olive oil
60ml/4 tbsp white wine vinegar
30ml/2 tbsp chopped fresh parsley
30ml/2 tbsp chopped fresh chives
30ml/2 tbsp chopped fresh tarragon or chervil
400g/14oz can haricot beans
400g/14oz can kidney beans
225g/8oz canned tuna in oil, drained and lightly flaked
parsley and chives, to garnish

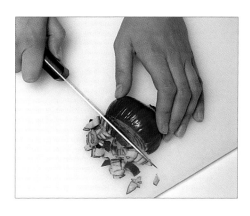

1 Finely chop the red onion, or the spring onions, if using.

—— COOK'S TIP ——

If you have problems with your hands, it is much easier to chop herbs with scissors rather than with a knife.

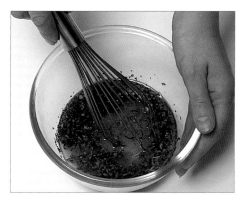

2 In a small bowl, beat together the mustard, oil, vinegar, parsley, chives and tarragon or chervil. Drain the canned haricot beans and kidney beans.

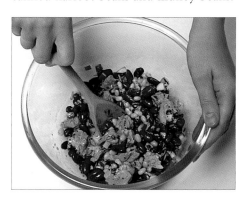

3 Mix together the red onion or spring onions, beans, flaked tuna and dressing in a large bowl. Toss well and serve, garnished with the extra parsley and whole chives.

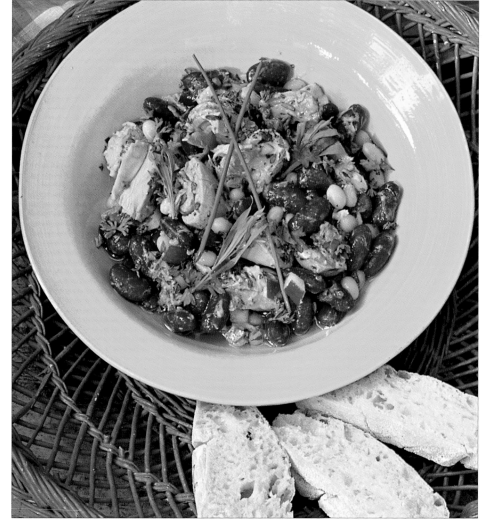

—— NUTRITION NOTES ——

Per portion:

Energy	774kcals/3173kJ
Fat, total	56.8g
saturated fat	8.2g
Protein	29.7g
Carbohydrate	38.6g
sugar, total	7.0g
Fibre – NSP	12.8g
Sodium	790mg

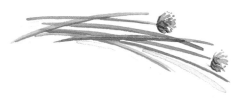

Stuffed Sardines

This Middle Eastern-inspired dish doesn't take a lot of preparation and is a meal in itself. Just serve with crisp green salad tossed in a fresh vinaigrette to make it complete.

INGREDIENTS

Serves 4

30ml/2 tbsp olive oil
75g/3oz/¾ cup wholemeal breadcrumbs or, if you are on a wheat-free diet, 2 small packets of plain potato crisps, crushed
50g/2oz/¼ cup sultanas
50g/2oz/½ cup pine nuts
1 onion, finely chopped or 15ml/1 tbsp dried onion
50g/2oz canned anchovy fillets, drained
60ml/4 tbsp chopped fresh parsley
900g/2lb fresh sardines, cleaned
salt and ground black pepper

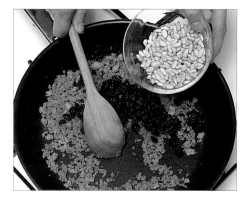

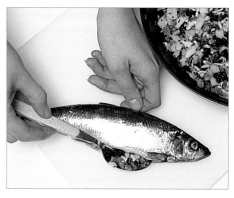

2 Add the sultanas, pine nuts, onion, anchovies, parsley and seasoning to the frying pan and mix well. If you are using crisps, instead of breacrumbs, mix all of the stuffing ingredients in a bowl.

3 Stuff each sardine with the mixture. Close the fish firmly and place them in a shallow ovenproof dish, closely packed together.

4 Scatter the remaining stuffing mixture over the sardines and bake for 30 minutes. Try serving this on a bed of salad leaves, and hand round lemon wedges, unless you are on a citrus-free diet in which case you could drizzle the dish with cider vinegar.

COOK'S TIP

If you find stuffing the sardines difficult, simply lay the fish in the baking dish and spread the stuffing over the top.

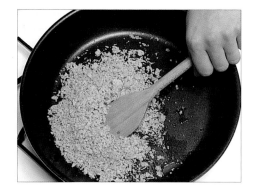

1 Preheat the oven to 200°C/400°F/ Gas 6. Heat the olive oil in a large frying pan and fry the breadcrumbs until crisp and golden.

NUTRITION NOTES

Per portion:

Energy	655kcals/2685kJ
Fat, total	37.7g
saturated fat	7.4g
Protein	54.2g
Carbohydrate	26.6g
sugar, total	11.7g
Fibre – NSP	1.4g
Sodium	907mg

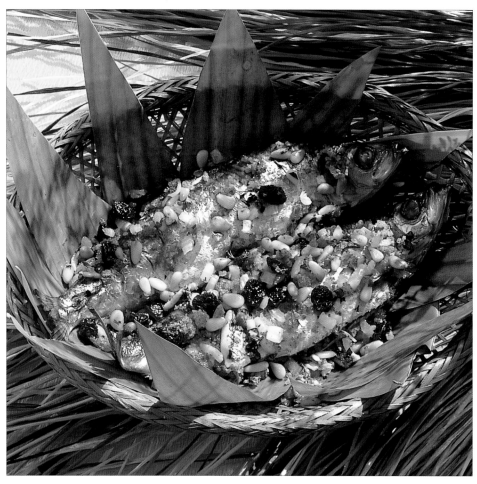

Rice Cakes with Smoked Salmon

Smoked salmon goes perfectly with these elegant rice cakes. Salmon is an oily fish, containing beneficial nutrients that work to reduce inflammation.

INGREDIENTS

Serves 4

15g/½oz/2 tbsp dried porcini mushrooms
30ml/2 tbsp olive oil
1 onion, chopped or 15ml/1 tbsp dried onion
225g/8oz/generous 1 cup risotto rice
about 90ml/6 tbsp white wine
about 750ml/1¼ pints/3 cups fish or chicken stock
15ml/1 tbsp chopped fresh parsley
15ml/1 tbsp snipped fresh chives
5ml/1 tsp chopped fresh dill
1 egg, lightly beaten
about 45ml/3 tbsp ground rice, plus extra for dusting
oil, for frying
175g/6oz smoked salmon, chopped
baby asparagus spears, roasted
salt and ground black pepper
60ml/4 tbsp soured cream or, if you are on a dairy-free diet, soya cream or coconut cream, to serve
radicchio and oakleaf salad, tossed in French dressing, to serve

---

NUTRITION NOTES

Per portion:

Energy	390kcals/1599kJ
Fat, total	12.9g
saturated fat	3.4g
Protein	18.5g
Carbohydrate	45.7g
sugar, total	2.8g
Fibre – NSP	0.5g
Sodium	852mg

VARIATION

If you have any risotto left from another recipe, use it to make the rice cakes.

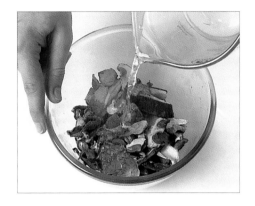

1 Place the porcini mushrooms in a bowl and cover with boiling water. Leave to soak for 15 minutes.

2 Heat the olive oil in a saucepan or frying pan and fry the onion for 3–4 minutes until soft.

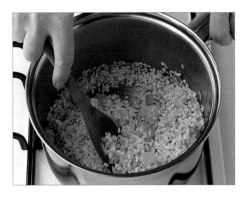

3 Add the rice to the pan and cook, stirring, for 3–4 minutes until the grains are thoroughly coated in oil. Pour in the wine and stock, a little at a time, stirring constantly over a gentle heat. Check that each quantity of liquid has been absorbed before adding more.

COOK'S TIPS

• If you would find it difficult to make the patties, omit the egg and the ground rice and cook the risotto for slightly longer. Top with spoonfuls of soured cream, soya cream or coconut cream and scatter the chopped smoked salmon over the top.
• Smoked salmon offcuts, available from most supermarkets, will be fine for this dish and are much cheaper.

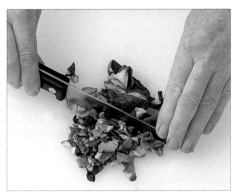

4 Drain the porcini mushrooms and chop them into small pieces. When the rice is tender, and all the liquid has been absorbed, stir in the mushrooms.

5 Add the parsley, chives, dill and seasoning to the risotto. Remove from the heat and set aside for a few minutes to cool. Add the beaten egg and mix well. Then stir in enough ground rice to bind the mixture – it should be soft but manageable.

6 Dust your hands with ground rice and shape the mixture into four patties, about 13cm/5in in diameter and about 2cm/¾in thick.

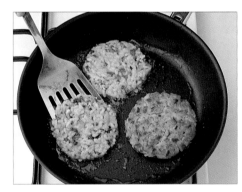

7 Heat the oil in a frying pan and fry the rice cakes, in batches if necessary, for 4–5 minutes until evenly browned on both sides. Drain on kitchen paper and cool slightly.

8 Place each rice cake on a plate and sprinkle over the chopped smoked salmon and asparagus spears. Serve with 15ml/1 tbsp soured cream, soya cream or coconut cream and a fresh salad.

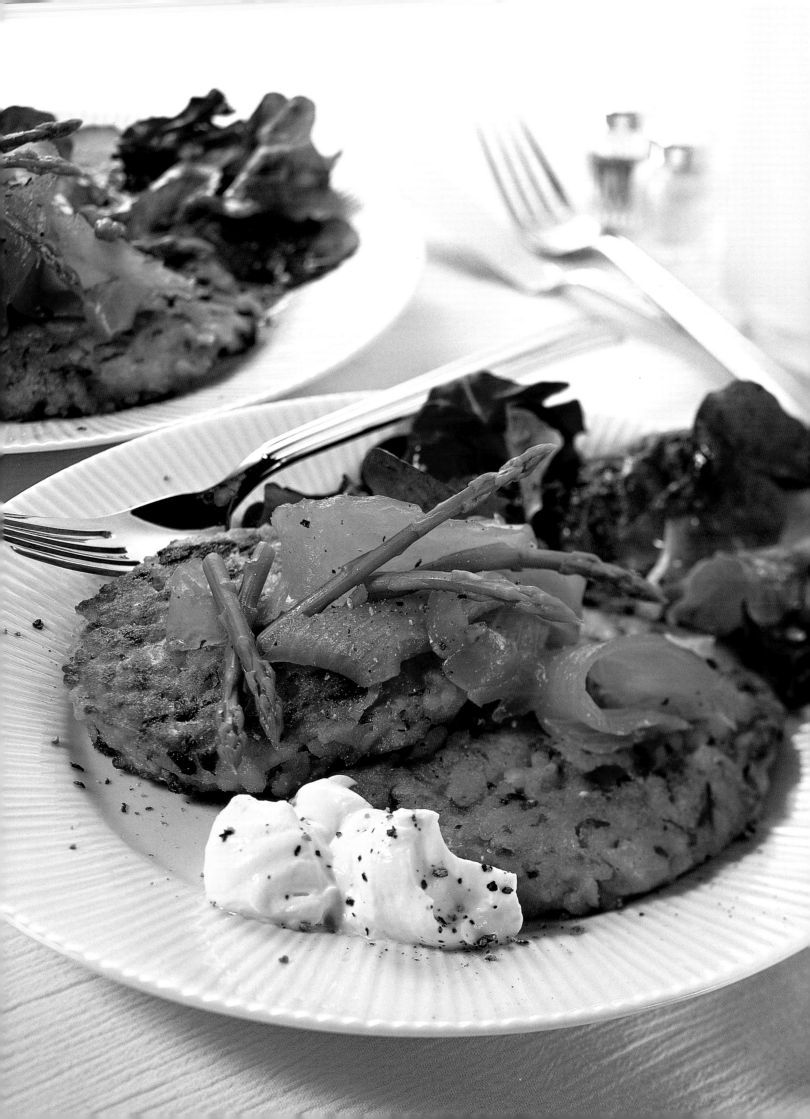

Sicilian Spaghetti with Sardines

This traditional dish is a great way to eat sardines, which are an excellent fish for building up your stock of anti-inflammatory alpha linolenic acid (ALA).

INGREDIENTS

Serves 4

12 fresh sardines, cleaned and boned
250ml/8fl oz/1 cup olive oil
1 onion or 15ml/1 tbsp dried onion
25g/1oz/¼ cup fresh dill, chopped
50g/2oz/½ cup pine nuts
25g/1oz/2 tbsp raisins, soaked in water
50g/2oz/½ cup fresh breadcrumbs or,
    if you are on a wheat-free diet,
    crushed plain potato crisps
450g/1lb spaghetti (wheat-free if you
    are on a wheat-free diet)
plain flour or, if you are on a wheat-free
    diet, potato or cornflour, for dusting
salt and ground black pepper

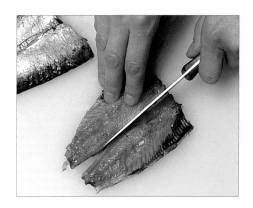

1 Wash the sardines and pat dry on kitchen paper. Open them out flat, then cut in half lengthways.

COOK'S TIP

If you have problems lifting heavy pans, place the spaghetti in a wire basket and cook in boiling water. You can lift out the spaghetti easily, and drain the water later, when cool.

2 Heat 30ml/2 tbsp of the oil in a pan. Chop the onion and fry until golden. Add the dill and cook gently for a minute or two. Add the pine nuts and raisins and season with salt and freshly ground black pepper to taste.

3 Meanwhile, place the breadcrumbs, if using, in a frying pan and dry fry until they are golden. Set aside.

4 Boil a large saucepan of salted water and add the spaghetti. Cook according to the instructions on the packet, until the spaghetti is *al dente*.

5 Heat the remaining oil in a pan. Dust the sardines with flour and fry in the hot oil for 2–3 minutes. Drain on kitchen paper.

6 Drain the spaghetti. Add the onion mixture and toss well. Transfer the spaghetti mixture to a serving platter and arrange the fried sardines on top. Sprinkle with the toasted breadcrumbs or crisps and serve immediately.

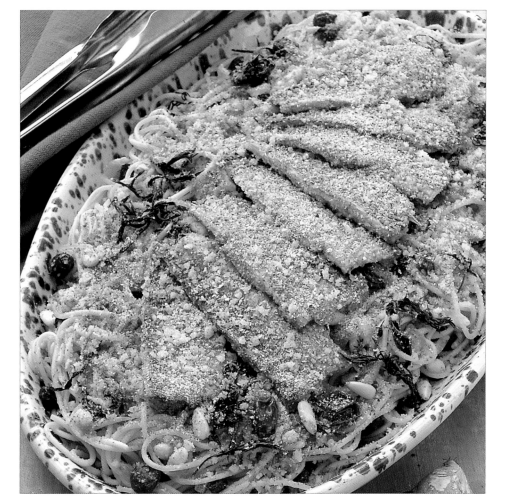

NUTRITION NOTES

Per portion:

Energy	1029kcals/4218kJ
Fat, total	62g
saturated fat	9.2g
Protein	31.3g
Carbohydrate	91.2g
sugar, total	10.6g
Fibre – NSP	4.2g
Sodium	98mg

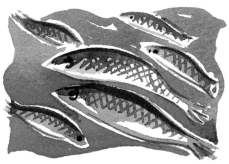

Barbecued Salmon with Red Onion Marmalade

The sweet, caramelized red onions provide the perfect contrast to the fish, in colour as well as flavour.

INGREDIENTS

Serves 4
4 salmon steaks, cut 2.5cm/1in thick
30ml/2 tbsp olive oil
salt and ground black pepper
fresh flat leaf parsley, to garnish

For the red onion marmalade
5 red onions, peeled
60ml/4 tbsp olive oil
175ml/6fl oz/¾ cup red wine vinegar
50ml/2fl oz/¼ cup crème de cassis
50ml/2fl oz/¼ cup grenadine
50ml/2fl oz/¼ cup red wine

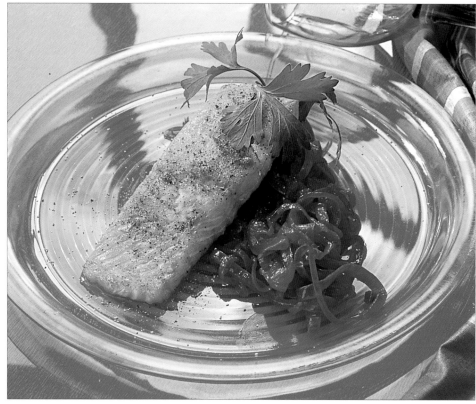

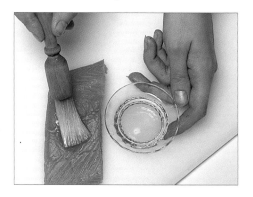

1 Brush the salmon steaks with the olive oil on both sides. Season the fish well with salt and ground black pepper.

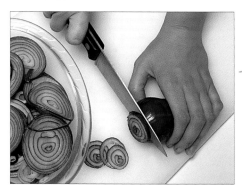

2 Finely slice the onions or chop them if that is easier. Heat the oil in a saucepan and add the onions. Sauté for 5 minutes.

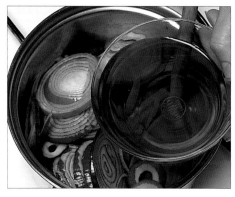

3 Stir in the remaining ingredients. Cook for about 10 minutes, or until the onions are glazed. Season well.

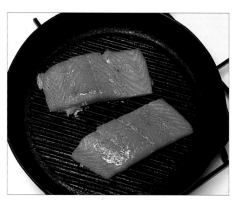

4 Brush the fish with a little more oil, and cook in a ridged grilling pan or on the barbecue for 4 minutes on either side. Transfer to warmed plates and garnish with parsley. Serve with the red onion marmalade.

NUTRITION NOTES

Per portion:

Energy	444kcals/1820kJ
Fat, total	30.2g
saturated fat	4.7g
Protein	25.3g
Carbohydrate	8.17g
sugar, total	8.17g
Fibre – NSP	0.0g
Sodium	57.1mg

COOK'S TIPS

• If you cannot find crème de cassis and grenadine, replace both of these ingredients with red wine instead.
• Fish cooks on barbecues well, but make sure it is at least 2.5cm/1in thick to make it easy to turn when cooking.

Salmon Risotto with Cucumber and Tarragon

An easy but tasty dish which can be served from the pot it was cooked in. Salmon is an oily fish, rich in ALA (alpha linolenic acid). This is beneficial to arthritis sufferers as it can help to reduce inflammation and joint pain.

INGREDIENTS

Serves 4

30ml/2 tbsp olive oil
small bunch of spring onions, white parts only, chopped with scissors
½ cucumber, peeled, seeded and chopped (see Cook's Tip)
350g/12oz/1¾ cups risotto rice
1.2 litres/2 pints/5 cups hot chicken or fish stock
150ml/¼ pint/⅔ cup dry white wine
450g/1lb salmon fillet, skinned and diced
45ml/3 tbsp chopped fresh tarragon
salt and ground black pepper

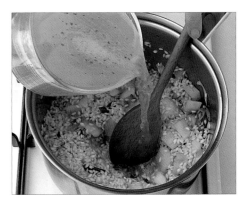

1 Heat the oil in a large saucepan or table-top cooker and add the spring onions and the cucumber. Cook for 2–3 minutes without allowing the spring onions to colour.

COOK'S TIP

If you would find peeling and seeding the cucumber difficult, just chop it with skin and seeds intact.

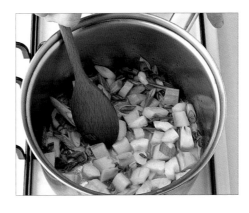

2 Stir in the rice, then add the stock and wine. Bring to the boil, then lower the heat and simmer, uncovered, for 10 minutes, stirring occasionally.

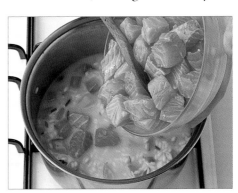

3 Stir in the diced salmon and season to taste with salt and ground black pepper. Continue cooking for a further 5 minutes, stirring occasionally, then switch off the heat. Cover and leave to stand for 5 minutes.

4 Remove the lid, add the chopped fresh tarragon and mix lightly to combine. Serve the risotto immediately, in warmed bowls.

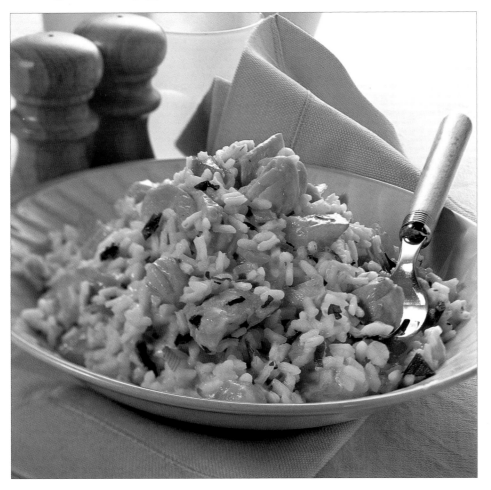

NUTRITION NOTES

Per portion:

Energy	606kcals/2484kJ
Fat, total	19.5g
saturated fat	2.9g
Protein	32.4g
Carbohydrate	66.9g
sugar, total	0.7g
Fibre – NSP	0.2g
Sodium	596mg

Roast Lamb with Spiced Apricot Stuffing

Cinnamon, cumin and apricots are complementary partners in a bulgur wheat stuffing used in this easy-to-carve joint.

INGREDIENTS

Serves 6

75g/3oz/½ cup bulgur wheat or, if you are on a wheat-free diet, brown rice (see Cook's Tips)
30ml/2 tbsp olive oil
1 small onion, finely chopped or 7.5ml/1½ tsp dried onion
1 garlic clove, crushed or 5ml/1 tsp garlic purée
5ml/1 tsp ground cinnamon
5ml/1 tsp ground cumin
175g/6oz/¾ cup chopped ready-to-eat dried apricots
50g/2oz/⅔ cup pine nuts
1 boned shoulder of lamb, about 1.75kg/4–4½ lb
120ml/4fl oz/½ cup red wine
120ml/4fl oz/½ cup lamb stock
salt and ground black pepper
fresh mint sprigs, to garnish

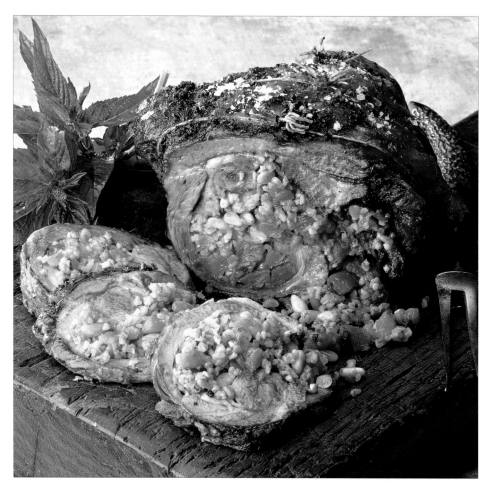

1 Place the bulgur wheat in a bowl and add sufficient warm water to cover. Leave to soak for 1 hour, then drain thoroughly.

2 Heat the oil in a saucepan. Add the onion and garlic and cook for about 5 minutes. Stir in the bulgur wheat, cinnamon, cumin, apricots and pine nuts and season to taste. Leave to cool.

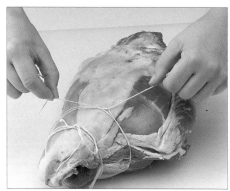

3 Preheat the oven to 180°C/350°F/ Gas 4. Open out the shoulder of lamb and spread the stuffing over. Roll it up firmly and tie tightly with string. Place in a roasting tin. Roast for 1 hour, then pour the red wine and stock into the roasting tin.

4 Roast the joint for 30 minutes more, then transfer to a heated plate, cover with foil and allow the meat to rest for 15–20 minutes before carving.

5 Meanwhile, skim the surface fat from the wine-flavoured stock in the roasting tin. Place the tin over a high heat and allow the gravy to bubble for a few minutes, stirring occasionally to incorporate any sediment. Carve the lamb neatly, arrange the slices on a serving platter and pour over the gravy. Serve at once, garnished with mint.

COOK'S TIPS

• If you are using brown rice, add it to the cooked onion and garlic at Step 2 with about 300ml/½ pint/1¼ cups stock. Bring to the boil; simmer until the rice is cooked. Then add the spices, apricots and pine nuts.
• If you would have problems stuffing and tying the lamb, leave it as a whole joint and roast for 40 minutes per kilogram, plus 20 minutes extra. Add the stock and wine halfway through, and cook the stuffing separately in a casserole.

NUTRITION NOTES

Per portion:

Energy	749kcals/3070kJ
Fat, total	52.5g
saturated fat	20.8g
Protein	44.8g
Carbohydrate	22.1g
sugar, total	11.7g
Fibre – NSP	2.3g
Sodium	272mg

Chicken with Mangetouts and Ginger

Ingredients

Serves 4

4 boned and skinned chicken breasts
225g/8oz mangetouts
45ml/3 tbsp olive oil
3 garlic cloves, finely chopped or
   10ml/2 tsp garlic purée
2.5cm/1in piece fresh root ginger,
   freshly grated or 10ml/2 tsp
   powdered ginger
5–6 spring onions, cut into 4cm/1½in
   lengths with scissors
10ml/2 tsp sesame oil
boiled rice, to serve; parsley, to garnish

For the marinade

5ml/1 tsp cornflour
15ml/1 tbsp light soy sauce, wheat-free
   if you are on a wheat-free diet
15ml/1 tbsp medium dry sherry
15ml/1 tbsp vegetable oil

For the sauce

5ml/1 tsp cornflour
10–15ml/2–3 tsp dark soy sauce, wheat-
   free if you are on a wheat-free diet
120ml/4fl oz/½ cup chicken stock
30ml/2 tbsp oyster sauce, or omit if
   you are on a wheat-free diet

1 Cut the chicken into thick strips. For the marinade, blend together the cornflour and soy sauce. Stir in the sherry and oil. Pour over the chicken, toss lightly, and leave for 30 minutes.

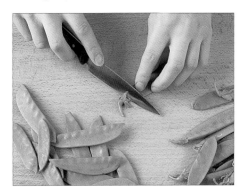

2 Trim the mangetouts and plunge into a pan of boiling salted water. Bring back to the boil and then drain and refresh under cold running water.

Cook's Tip

If you have trouble with your hands, put the mangetouts into a sieve. Fill a pan with water, bring to the boil, then lower in the sieve with the mangetouts for 1 minute. Remove and refresh under cold running water.

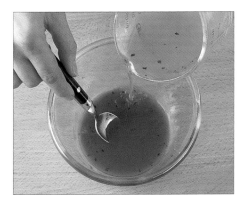

3 To make the sauce, mix together the cornflour, soy sauce, stock and oyster sauce and set aside.

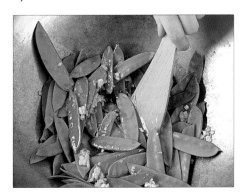

4 Heat 15ml/1 tbsp of the olive oil in a wok and add the garlic, ginger and spring onions. Stir-fry for 30 seconds. Add the chicken with its marinade, and cook briskly for a couple of minutes. Lower the heat, cover the wok and simmer for 15 minutes or until the chicken pieces are cooked through. Stir in the sesame oil, the sauce and the mangetouts. Cook for a further couple of minutes. Serve with boiled rice and garnish with parsley.

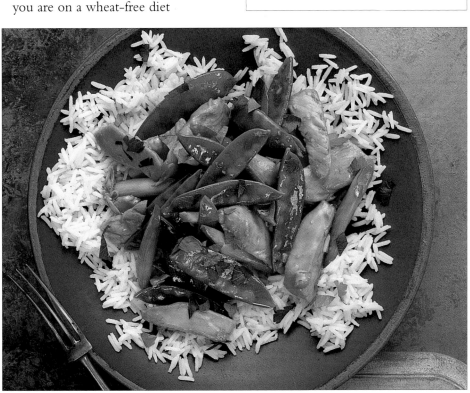

Nutrition Notes

Per portion:

Energy	290kcals/1189kJ
Fat, total	13.7g
saturated fat	2.0g
Protein	38.9g
Carbohydrate	3.1g
sugar, total	2.3g
Fibre – NSP	1.6g
Sodium	306mg

Chicken with Beans

This substantial casserole is bursting with flavour, texture and colour.

INGREDIENTS

Serves 4

275g/10oz dried kidney or other beans, soaked overnight then cooked in fast boiling water for 20 minutes, or 400g/14oz can kidney beans, drained
8 chicken portions, such as thighs and drumsticks
12 bacon rashers, rind removed
2 large onions, thinly sliced or 30ml/ 2 tbsp dried onion
250ml/8fl oz/1 cup dry white wine
2.5ml/½ tsp chopped fresh sage or oregano, or 1.5ml/¼ tsp dried
2.5ml/½ tsp chopped fresh rosemary, or 1.5ml/¼ tsp dried
generous pinch of grated nutmeg
150ml/¼ pint/⅔ cup soured cream or, if you are on a dairy-free diet, plain dairy-free yogurt
15ml/1 tbsp chilli powder or, if you are on a solanacae-free diet, ground ginger
salt and ground black pepper
sprigs of rosemary, to garnish
lemon wedges, to serve (optional)

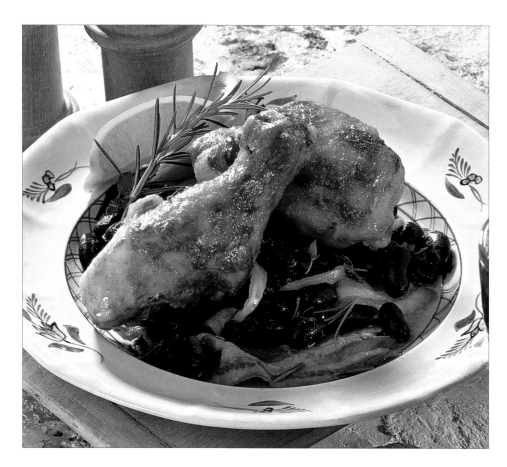

1 Rinse and drain the beans well and trim the chicken pieces. Season the chicken with salt and pepper.

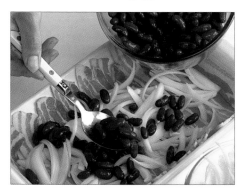

2 Arrange the bacon around the sides and base of an ovenproof dish. Sprinkle over half the sliced onion and then half the kidney beans, followed by another layer of onion and then the remaining beans.

3 Preheat the oven to 180°C/350°F/ Gas 4. Pour the wine into a large bowl and add the sage or oregano, rosemary and nutmeg. Mix the wine and the herbs together and then pour over the layers of onion and beans in the dish.

4 In another bowl, mix together the soured cream or dairy-free yogurt and the chilli powder or ground ginger.

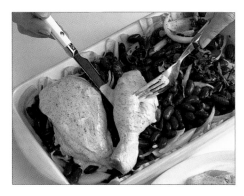

5 Toss the chicken in the soured cream or yogurt mixture, and place on top of the beans.

6 Cover with foil and bake in the oven for 1¼–1½ hours, removing the foil for the last 15 minutes of cooking. Garnish with rosemary and serve with the lemon wedges, if using.

COOK'S TIP

Kidney beans are very nutritious, but it is essential to cook the dried ones in fast boiling water for 20 minutes, in order to kill the toxins they contain.

NUTRITION NOTES

Per portion:

Energy	665kcals/2726kJ
Fat, total	31.9g
saturated fat	12.2g
Protein	57.5g
Carbohydrate	29.0g
sugar, total	12.1g
Fibre – NSP	7.8g
Sodium	1531mg

Stuffed Fennel

Fennel not only tastes delicious but it divides into neat boat shapes, ideal for stuffing.

INGREDIENTS

Serves 4
2 large bulbs fennel
3 eggs
30ml/2 tbsp olive oil
1 onion, chopped or 15ml/1 tbsp dried onion
2 chicken breasts, skinned and boned
225g/8oz/2½ cups trimmed and chopped oyster mushrooms
60ml/4 tbsp plain flour or, if you are on a wheat-free diet, potato or cornflour
300ml/½ pint/1¼ cups home-made or canned chicken broth, boiling
5ml/1 tsp Dijon mustard
30ml/2 tbsp sherry
salt and ground black pepper
fresh parsley sprigs, to garnish
boiled rice, to serve

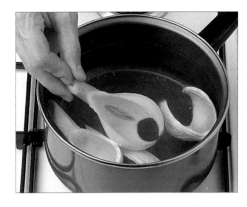

1 Preheat the oven to 190°C/375°F/ Gas 5. Trim the base of the fennel and pull each bulb apart into four pieces (save the central part). Boil the fennel in salted water for 3–4 minutes, then drain and leave to cool. Boil the eggs for 10 minutes. Allow to cool, then peel and set aside.

2 Finely chop the central part of the fennel. Sauté gently in oil with the onion for 3–4 minutes.

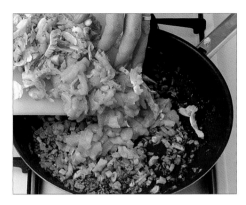

3 Cut the chicken into pieces and add to the frying pan with the mushrooms. Cook over a moderate heat for 6 minutes, stirring frequently. Add the flour, potato or cornflour and remove from the heat.

4 Gradually add the chicken broth, making sure the thickener is completely absorbed. Return to the heat and simmer until thickened, stirring all the time. Chop one of the eggs into the chicken mixture, add the mustard, sherry and seasoning to taste.

5 Arrange the fennel in a baking dish. Spoon the filling into each one, cover with foil and bake for 20–25 minutes. Serve on a bed of rice, garnished with the remaining eggs, quartered; and parsley.

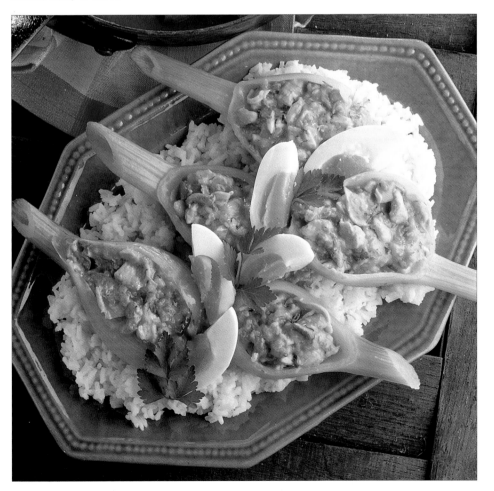

NUTRITION NOTES

Per portion:

Energy	91kcals/373kJ
Fat, total	6.0g
saturated fat	0.8g
Protein	2.8g
Carbohydrate	4.8g
sugar, total	3.6g
Fibre – NSP	2.9g
Sodium	193mg

COOK'S TIP

If you find the fennel difficult to cut, cook it before trying to cut it. It will be much easier to deal with once it is cooked.

Glazed Sweet Potatoes with Bacon

Smoky bacon is the perfect addition to these melt-in-the-mouth sugar-topped potatoes. This is a good basic dish if you are on a solanacae-free diet.

INGREDIENTS

Serves 4

oil, for greasing
900g/2lb sweet potatoes
115g/4oz/½ cup soft light brown sugar
30ml/2 tbsp lemon juice or, if you are on a citrus-free diet, 30ml/2 tbsp cider vinegar
45ml/3 tbsp olive oil
4 strips smoked lean bacon, cut into matchsticks
salt and ground black pepper
chopped flat leaf parsley, to garnish

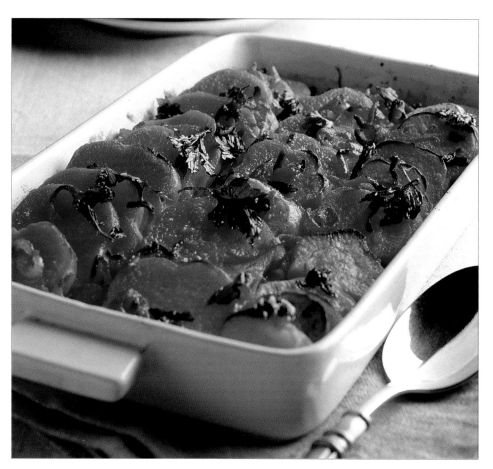

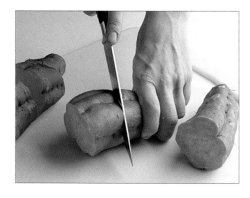

1 Preheat the oven to 190°C/375°F/ Gas 5 and lightly oil a shallow ovenproof dish. Cut each unpeeled sweet potato crosswise into three pieces and steam for about 25 minutes until they are just tender. Leave the sweet potatoes to cool.

NUTRITION NOTES

Per portion:

Energy	378kcals/1549kJ
Fat, total	7.5g
saturated fat	2.1g
Protein	6.8g
Carbohydrate	77.0g
sugar, total	41.9g
Fibre – NSP	5.4g
Sodium	483mg

2 When the potatoes are cool enough to handle, peel and slice thickly.

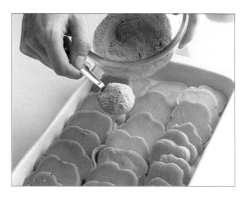

3 Arrange the potatoes in a single layer, overlapping the slices, in the prepared dish. Sprinkle the sugar over the top of the sweet potatoes.

COOK'S TIP

If you find it too fiddly to use a knife to cut the bacon into matchsticks, try using scissors instead.

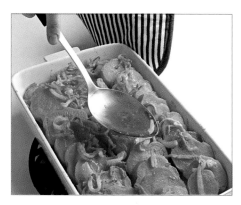

4 Lightly sprinkle over the lemon juice or cider vinegar and drizzle with oil. Top the sweet potatoes with the bacon and season with salt and freshly ground black pepper to taste. Bake uncovered for 35–40 minutes, basting once or twice.

5 Preheat the grill to a high heat. Sprinkle the potatoes with parsley. Place under the grill for 2–3 minutes until the potatoes are browned and the bacon is crispy. Serve hot.

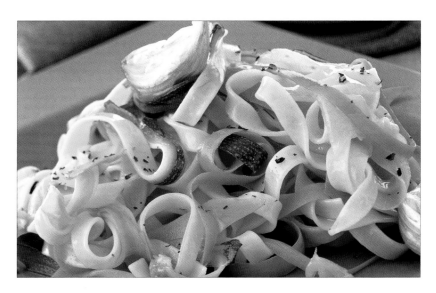

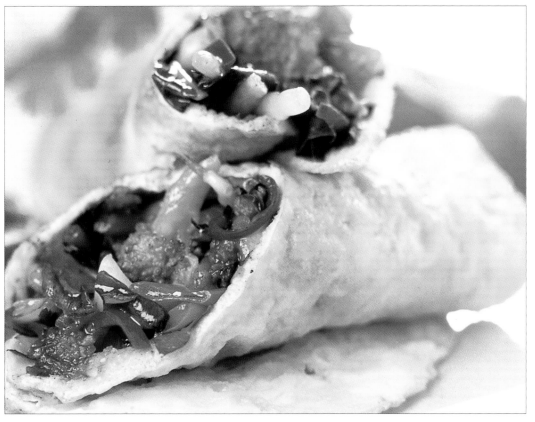

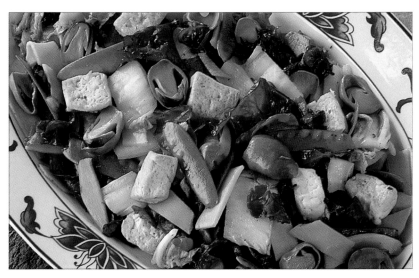

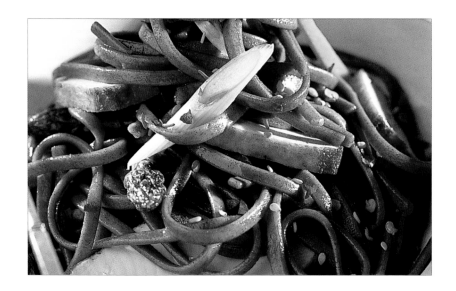

VEGETARIAN DISHES

This delicious selection of recipes includes dishes that use familiar

vegetables, such as the courgettes and carrots in Three Colour

Tagliatelle, and others that encourage you to experiment with different

ingredients. Try chard leaves in a traditional French omelette or make

the tasty Jerusalem Artichoke Risotto.

The recipes in this section are nutritious, fairly easy to prepare, and

follow the guidelines for a low-fat meat-free diet.

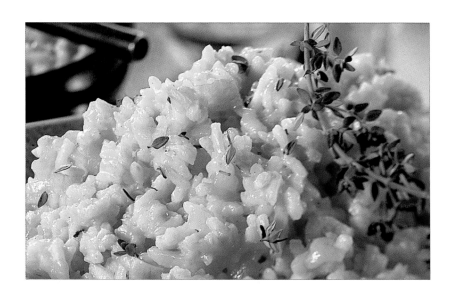

Three Colour Tagliatelle

This attractive dish might look difficult to prepare, but the colourful vegetable "ribbons" are far easier to cut than you would think.

INGREDIENTS

Serves 4

2 large courgettes
2 large carrots
250g/9oz fresh tagliatelle, wheat-free if you are on a wheat-free diet
60ml/4 tbsp extra virgin olive oil
flesh of 2 roasted garlic cloves, plus extra roasted garlic cloves, to serve (optional), or 10ml/2 tsp crushed raw garlic or garlic purée
salt and ground black pepper
30ml/2 tbsp toasted sunflower seeds, to serve (optional)

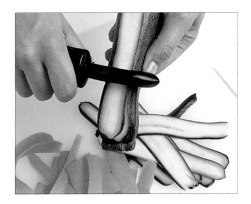

1 Using a vegetable peeler, cut the courgettes and carrots into long thin ribbons.

2 Bring a large pan of salted water to the boil. Put the carrots and courgette ribbons into a sieve. Sink them into the boiling water. Bring the water back to the boil and boil for 30 seconds, then remove and set aside.

3 Cook the pasta according to the instructions on the packet, until it is *al dente*. You may prefer to cook it in a wire basket. That way, you can lift out the food easily, and empty the heavy pan of water when it is cool.

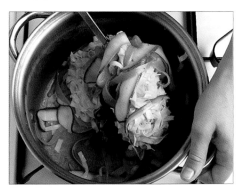

4 Drain the pasta and return it to the pan. Add the vegetable ribbons, oil, garlic and seasoning and toss over a medium to high heat until the pasta and vegetables are glistening with oil. Serve immediately, with extra roasted garlic and sunflower seeds, if you like.

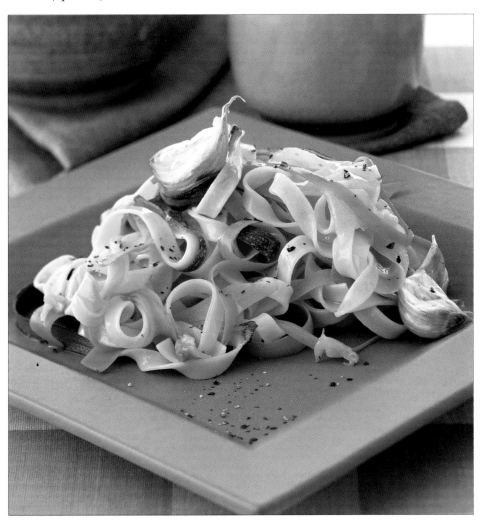

COOK'S TIPS

• To roast garlic, put a whole head of garlic on a lightly oiled baking sheet. Place in an oven preheated to 180°C/350°F/Gas 4 and roast for about 30 minutes. Remove the garlic from the oven and set aside. When cool enough to handle, dig out the flesh from the cloves with a small, sharp spoon.
• If you are struggling with the vegetable peeler, use more courgettes, which are easier to prepare, and fewer carrots.

NUTRITION NOTES

Per portion:

Energy	240kcals/984kJ
Fat, total	15.4g
saturated fat	2.09g
Protein	5.05g
Carbohydrate	21.7g
sugar, total	6.4g
Fibre – NSP	2.3g
Sodium	49mg

Braised Chinese Vegetables

The original recipe calls for no less than 18 different ingredients to represent the 18 Buddhas, but nowadays four to six items are regarded as quite sufficient.

INGREDIENTS

Serves 4

10g/¼oz dried black fungus (wood-ears)
75g/3oz straw mushrooms, drained
75g/3oz sliced bamboo shoots, drained
50g/2oz mangetouts
115g/4oz beancurd (tofu)
175g/6oz Chinese leaves
45–60ml/3–4 tbsp vegetable oil
5ml/1 tsp salt
2.5ml/½ tsp light brown sugar
15ml/1 tbsp light soy sauce, which should be wheat-free tamari if you are on a wheat-free diet
few drops sesame oil (optional)
30ml/2 tbsp pumpkin seeds (optional)

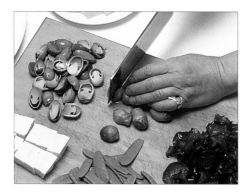

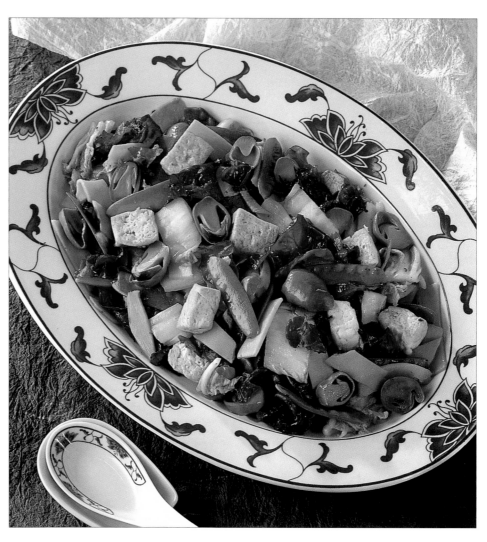

1 Soak the black fungus (wood-ears) in cold water for 20–25 minutes, then rinse and discard the hard stalks, if any. Cut the straw mushrooms in half lengthways, if large – keep them whole, if small. Rinse and drain the bamboo shoot slices. Top and tail the mangetouts. Cut the beancurd into about 12 small pieces. Cut the Chinese leaves into small pieces about the same size as the mangetouts.

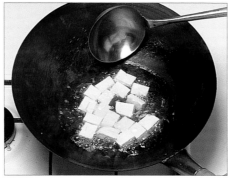

2 Harden the beancurd pieces by placing them in a wok or saucepan of boiling water for about 2 minutes. Remove with a slotted spoon and drain.

3 Heat the oil in the wok or saucepan and lightly brown the beancurd pieces on both sides. Remove with a slotted spoon and keep warm.

4 Stir-fry all the vegetables in the wok or saucepan for about 1½ minutes, then add the beancurd pieces, salt, sugar and soy sauce. Continue stirring for another minute, then cover and braise for 2–3 minutes. Sprinkle with sesame oil and pumpkin seeds, if using, and serve immediately.

COOK'S TIP

Remember that you can use scissors to cut up all the ingredients if you find it easier.

— NUTRITION NOTES —

Per portion:

Energy	126kcals/516kJ
Fat, total	10.6g
saturated fat	1.4g
Protein	5.6g
Carbohydrate	2.0g
sugar, total	1.6g
Fibre – NSP	1.3g
Sodium	274mg

Coriander Omelette Parcels with Vegetables

These exotic egg rolls are packed with antioxidants such as vitamins C and E, while ginger is well known for its anti-inflammatory properties.

INGREDIENTS

Serves 4

130g/4½oz broccoli, cut into
   small florets
30ml/2 tbsp groundnut oil
1cm/½in piece fresh root ginger, finely
   grated or 5ml/1 tsp ginger purée or
   5ml/1 tsp powdered ginger
1 large garlic clove, crushed or 5ml/
   1 tsp garlic purée
2 red chillies, seeded and finely sliced, or
   omit if you are on a solanacae-free diet
4 spring onions, sliced diagonally
175g/6oz/3 cups shredded pak choi
50g/2oz/2 cups fresh coriander leaves,
   plus extra to garnish
115g/4oz/½ cup beansprouts
45ml/3 tbsp black bean sauce, wheat-
   free if you are on a wheat-free diet
4 eggs
salt and freshly ground black pepper

1 Put the broccoli florets in the top of a steamer, submerge them in boiling water for 2 minutes, remove, then refresh under cold running water.

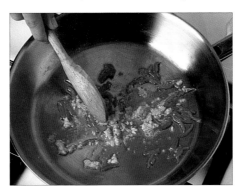

2 Meanwhile, heat 15ml/1 tbsp of the oil in a frying pan or wok. Add the ginger, garlic and half the chilli, if using, and stir-fry for 1 minute.

3 Add the spring onions, broccoli and pak choi to the pan or wok, and stir-fry for about 2 minutes more, tossing the vegetables continuously to prevent sticking and to cook evenly. Roughly chop three-quarters of the coriander and add.

4 Add the beansprouts and stir-fry for 1 minute, then add the black bean sauce and heat through for 1 minute. Remove from the heat. Keep warm.

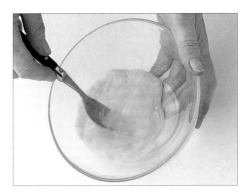

5 Whisk the eggs and season well. Heat a little oil in a frying pan and add a quarter of the beaten egg. Swirl over the base of the pan, then add a quarter of the remaining coriander leaves. Cook the omelette until set. Turn out and keep warm. Make three more omelettes. Add more oil when necessary.

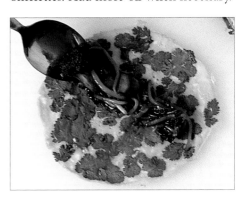

6 Spoon the stir-fry on to the omelettes, roll up and cut in half. Garnish with coriander leaves and chilli.

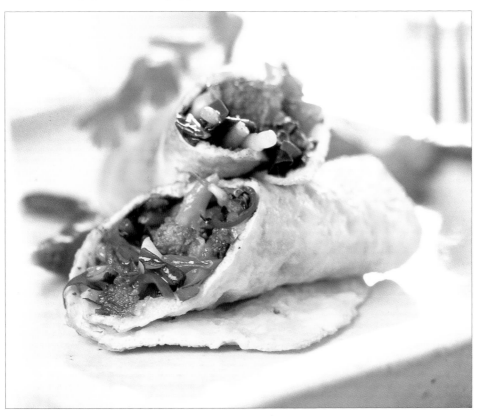

NUTRITION NOTES	
Per portion:	
Energy	150kcals/615kJ
Fat, total	11.5g
saturated fat	2.7g
Protein	9.0g
Carbohydrate	2.7g
sugar, total	2.4g
Fibre – NSP	1.7g
Sodium	327mg

Teriyaki Soba Noodles with Asparagus

You can, of course, buy ready-made teriyaki sauce, but it is easy to prepare at home using ingredients that are now readily available in supermarkets and Asian shops. Japanese soba noodles are made from buckwheat flour, which gives them a unique texture and colour, and makes them suitable for those on wheat-free diets!

INGREDIENTS

Serves 4

15ml/1 tbsp sesame seeds
350g/12oz soba noodles
30ml/2 tbsp sesame oil
200g/7oz asparagus tips
30ml/2 tbsp groundnut or vegetable oil
225g/8oz block of beancurd (tofu)
2 spring onions, cut diagonally
1 carrot, cut into matchsticks (optional)
2.5ml/½ tsp chilli flakes or omit if on a
   solanacae-free diet
salt and ground black pepper

For the teriyaki sauce
60ml/4 tbsp dark soy sauce, wheat-free
   if you are on a wheat-free diet
60ml/4 tbsp Japanese sake or dry sherry
60ml/4 tbsp mirin, wheat-free if you
   are on a wheat-free diet
5ml/1 tsp caster sugar

NUTRITION NOTES	
Per portion:	
Energy	492kcals/2017kJ
Fat, total	16.8g
saturated fat	2.0g
Protein	13.4g
Carbohydrate	72.1g
sugar, total	6.1g
Fibre – NSP	4.3g
Sodium	871mg

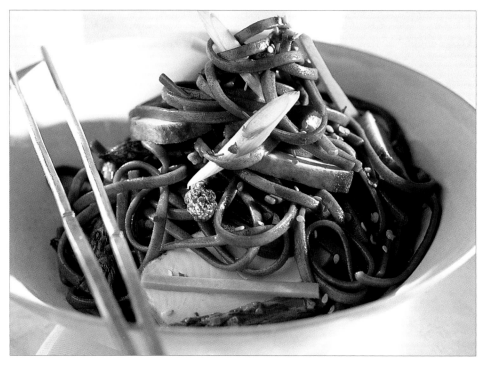

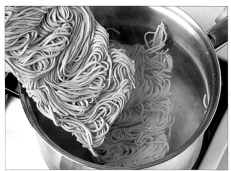

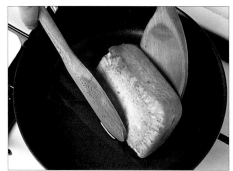

1 Toast the sesame seeds in a dry frying pan over a medium heat for 2 minutes, tossing frequently. Set aside.

2 Cook the noodles according to the instructions on the packet, then drain and rinse under cold running water. Set aside.

3 Heat the sesame oil in a ridged grilling pan or in a baking tray placed under the grill until very hot. Turn down the heat to medium, then cook the asparagus for 8–10 minutes, turning frequently, until tender and browned. Set aside.

HEALTH BENEFITS

Sesame seeds are an excellent source of the antioxidant vitamin E, which acts as a natural preservative, preventing oxidation and strengthening the heart and nerves.

4 Meanwhile, heat the oil in a frying pan, wok or table-top cooker until very hot. Add the beancurd and fry for 8–10 minutes until golden, turning it occasionally to crisp all sides. Remove from the pan and leave to drain on kitchen paper. Cut into 1cm/½in slices.

5 To prepare the teriyaki sauce, mix all of the ingredients together, then pour into a frying pan, wok or table-top cooker and heat gently.

6 Toss in the noodles and stir. Heat through for 1–2 minutes, then spoon into warmed serving bowls with the beancurd and asparagus. Scatter with spring onions, and the carrot and chilli flakes, if using them. Season, then add the sesame seeds and serve.

Beancurd and Crunchy Vegetables

You might like to add sunflower seeds to this, as they contain the anti-inflammatory acid, GLA.

INGREDIENTS

Serves 4

2 × 225g/8oz blocks smoked beancurd (tofu), cubed
45ml/3 tbsp soy sauce or, if you are on a wheat-free diet, tamari
30ml/2 tbsp dry sherry or vermouth
15ml/1 tbsp sesame oil, plus extra to serve (optional)
45ml/3 tbsp groundnut or sunflower oil
2 leeks, thinly sliced
2 carrots, cut in sticks
1 large courgette, thinly sliced
115g/4oz baby sweetcorn, halved
115g/4oz button or shiitake mushrooms, sliced
15ml/1 tbsp sesame seeds
1 packet of noodles, cooked, or, if you are on a wheat-free diet, rice noodles or wheat-free pasta

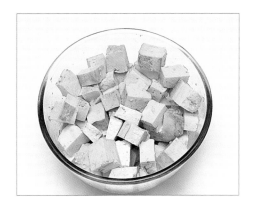

1 Marinate the beancurd (tofu) in the soy sauce, sherry or vermouth and sesame oil for at least half an hour. Drain and reserve the marinade.

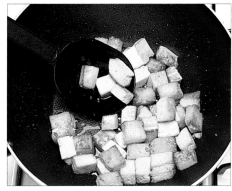

2 Heat the groundnut or sunflower oil in a wok or table-top cooker and stir-fry the beancurd cubes until they are browned all over. Remove and reserve.

VARIATION

Beancurd (tofu) is also excellent marinated and threaded on to small skewers, then lightly grilled or cooked on a barbecue. Serve the beancurd with pitta bread and a green salad.

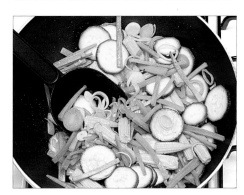

3 Stir-fry the leeks, carrots, courgette and baby corn, for about 2 minutes. Add the sliced mushrooms and cook for a further minute.

4 Return the beancurd to the wok and pour in the marinade. Heat until bubbling, then scatter over the sesame seeds. Serve as soon as possible with the hot cooked noodles or pasta, dressed in a little sesame oil, if liked.

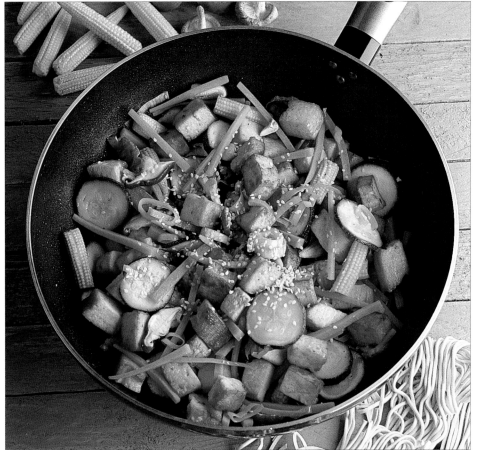

NUTRITION NOTES	
Per portion:	
Energy	425kcals/1742kJ
Fat, total	20.8g
saturated fat	4.0g
Protein	18.6g
Carbohydrate	41.2g
sugar, total	5.1g
Fibre – NSP	3.4g
Sodium	520mg

Butter Bean and Pesto Pasta

This rich and creamy pasta dish is simplicity itself to make, and yet it tastes sensational.

INGREDIENTS

Serves 4

225g/8oz pasta shapes, wheat-free if
  you are on a wheat-free diet
fresh nutmeg, grated
30ml/2 tbsp extra virgin olive oil
400g/14oz can butter beans, drained
45ml/3 tbsp pesto sauce but see Cook's
  Tip if you are on a dairy-free diet
150ml/¼ pint/⅔ cup single cream or,
  if you are on a dairy-free diet, soya
  cream or dairy-free plain yogurt
salt and ground black pepper

To serve

45ml/3 tbsp pine nuts
cheese, grated (optional), omit if on a
  dairy-free diet
sprigs of fresh basil, to garnish (optional)

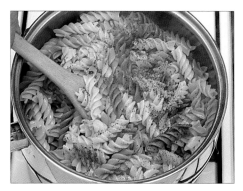

1 Boil the pasta in a large saucepan until it is *al dente*, then drain, leaving it a little wet. Return the pasta to the pan, season, and stir in the grated nutmeg and olive oil.

COOK'S TIP

Most pesto contains Parmesan cheese which should be avoided if you are on a dairy-free diet. If you cannot find a ready-made pesto that is suitable for your diet, it is easy to make your own. Follow a recipe for making pesto, substituting a hard sheep's milk cheese such as Pecorino for the Parmesan.

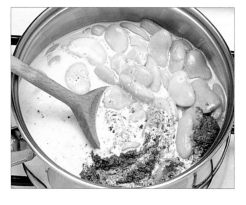

2 Heat the beans in a saucepan with the pesto and cream or yogurt, stirring the mixture until it begins to simmer. Toss the beans and pesto into the pasta and mix well.

3 Serve the pasta in bowls and top with pine nuts and a little grated cheese if you wish. Garnish with basil sprigs, if liked, and serve immediately.

NUTRITION NOTES

Per portion:

Energy	528kcals/2164kJ
Fat, total	27.2g
saturated fat	7.4g
Protein	17.5g
Carbohydrate	56.8g
sugar, total	5.1g
Fibre – NSP	6.4g
Sodium	494mg

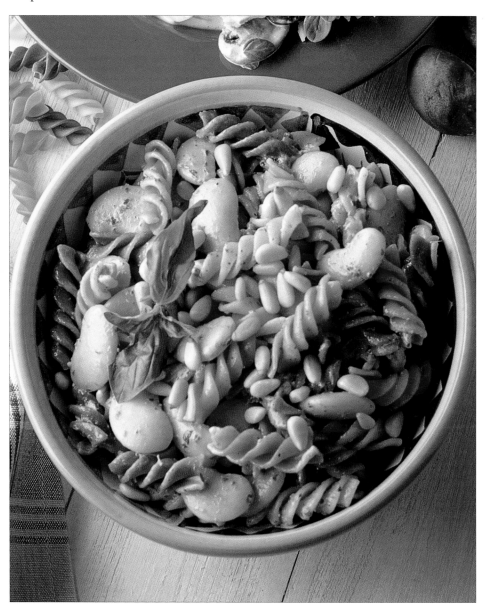

Mushroom and Sunflower Seed Flan

The flan can be prepared in advance and is good warm or cold. Spinach is an excellent source of antioxidants, which protect against cancer, as well as minimizing the joint damage caused by arthritis.

INGREDIENTS

Serves 4
150g/5oz/1 cup wholewheat flour or, if you are on a wheat-free diet, 75g/3oz/½ cup gram or chick-pea flour plus 75g/3oz/½ cup rice flour
75g/3oz butter or dairy-free spread
45ml/3 tbsp walnut or sunflower oil
175g/5oz fresh baby sweetcorn
50g/2oz sunflower seeds
225g/7oz button mushrooms, wiped
75g/3oz fresh spinach or defrosted frozen leaf spinach
juice 1 lemon or, if you are on a citrus-free diet, 30ml/2 tbsp cider vinegar
salt and ground black pepper

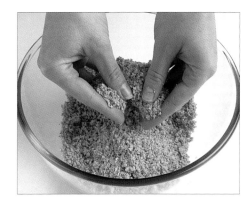

1 Heat the oven to 180°C/350°F/ Gas 4. Make the pastry by rubbing the butter or spread into the flour.

2 Add enough water to make a firm dough. Roll it out and line a 23–25cm/9–10in flan dish. You can press the pastry out into the flan dish rather than rolling it if you have problems with your hands. This may also be easier if you are using wheat-free flours, which make crumbly pastry.

3 Prick the bottom of the pastry case, line it with foil, and weight it with beans or rice. Bake for 10 minutes with the foil, then 10 minutes without, so that the pastry case becomes crisp.

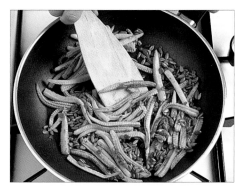

4 Heat the oil in a pan and add the corn and sunflower seeds. Fry briskly till they are browned all over.

5 Add the mushrooms, reduce the heat slightly and cook for about 3 minutes. Add the chopped spinach, stir well, cover the pan and cook for a further couple of minutes.

6 Add the lemon juice or vinegar and season well. Make sure the ingredients are well amalgamated, then spoon them into the flan case. Serve the flan at once, or, if you prefer, leave to cool and serve at room temperature.

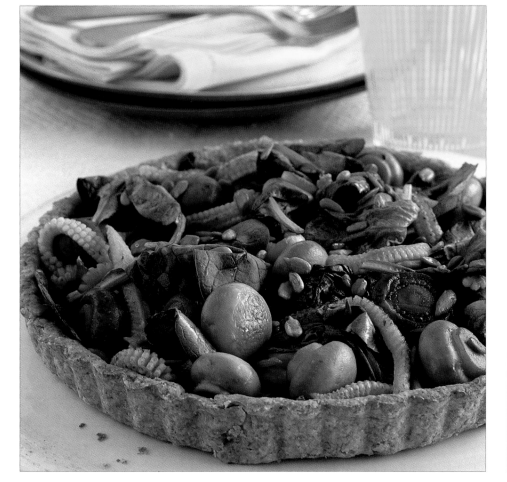

COOK'S TIP

If your hands are stiff and painful, combine the fat and flour in a food processor.

NUTRITION NOTES

Per portion:

Energy	447kcals/1837kJ
Fat, total	32.0g
saturated fat	11.7g
Protein	12.5g
Carbohydrate	28.8g
sugar, total	2.5g
Fibre – NSP	4.6g
Sodium	401mg

Jerusalem Artichoke Risotto

The delicious and distinctive flavour of Jerusalem artichokes makes this simple and warming risotto something special.

INGREDIENTS

Serves 4

400g/14oz Jerusalem artichokes
60ml/4 tbsp olive oil
1 onion, finely chopped or 15ml/1 tbsp dried onion
1 garlic clove, crushed or 5ml/1 tsp puréed garlic
275g/10oz/1½ cups risotto rice
120ml/4fl oz/½ cup fruity white wine
1 litre/1¾ pints/4 cups simmering vegetable stock
10ml/2 tsp chopped fresh thyme
40g/1½oz/½ cup freshly grated Parmesan cheese, plus extra to serve, or, if you are on a dairy-free diet, 40g/1½oz chopped black olives
salt and ground black pepper
fresh thyme sprigs, to garnish

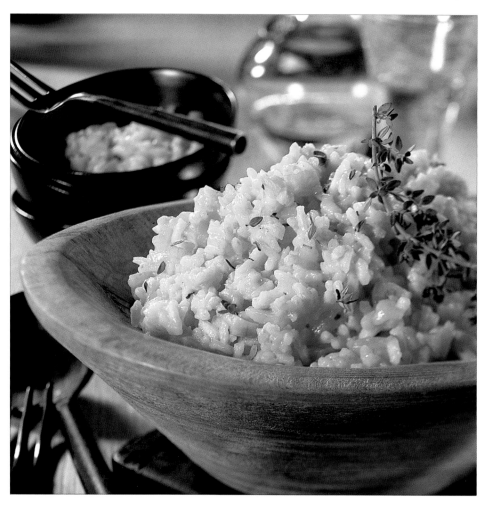

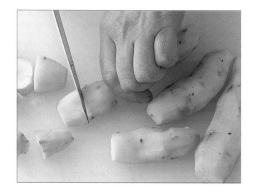

1 Peel the artichokes, cut them into pieces and steam over boiling water. Mash them with a potato masher or purée them in a bowl with a hand-held blender. Add 15ml/1 tbsp olive oil and season with salt.

COOK'S TIP

If you find the artichokes difficult to peel, scrub them well and cook them without peeling. It will be much easier to remove the nobbles when they are cooked.

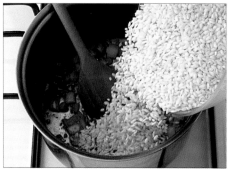

2 Heat the remaining oil in a pan and fry the onion and garlic for 5–6 minutes until soft. Add the rice and cook for about 2 minutes, or until the grains are translucent around the edges.

3 Pour in the wine, stir until it has been absorbed, then add the stock, a ladleful at a time, with each quantity absorbed before adding more. When you have one ladleful of stock left, stir in the artichokes and the thyme.

4 Continue cooking until the risotto is creamy and the artichokes are hot. Stir in the Parmesan or black olives and season to taste.

5 Remove the risotto from the heat, cover the pan and leave to stand for a few minutes. Serve garnished with thyme and sprinkled with Parmesan cheese, if using.

NUTRITION NOTES

Per portion:

Energy	483kcals/1980kJ
Fat, total	16.7g
saturated fat	3.7g
Protein	13.2g
Carbohydrate	65.6g
sugar, total	3.8g
Fibre – NSP	4.2g
Sodium	701mg

Red Onion and Broccoli Risotto

INGREDIENTS

Serves 4
30ml/2 tbsp olive oil

2 red onions, finely sliced or 30ml/
2 tbsp dried onion

2 garlic cloves, finely sliced or 5ml/
1 tsp garlic purée

150g/5oz risotto rice

300ml/½ pint/1¼ cups dry white wine

600ml/1 pint/2½ cups water

200g/7oz broccoli florets, steamed for a
few minutes until partially cooked

250g/9oz smoked or marinated
beancurd (tofu), cubed

200g/7oz can water chestnuts, drained
and halved

50g/2oz roasted salted cashew nuts

salt and ground black pepper

1 Heat the oil in a large pan. Gently
cook the onion and garlic until soft.

2 Add the rice, wine and water,
stirring gently. Bring to a simmer
and cook for 10–15 minutes or until
the rice is soft and the liquid has been
absorbed. Add more liquid if necessary.

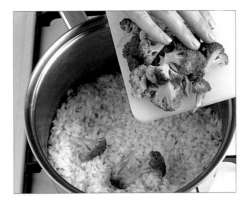

3 Add the broccoli florets, beancurd
(tofu), water chestnuts and cashew
nuts to the rice. Mix well and season
with salt and pepper to taste. Serve the
risotto warm or cold.

—— NUTRITION NOTES ——
Per portion:

Energy	365kcals/1496kJ
Fat, total	15.6g
saturated fat	2.4g
Protein	14.3g
Carbohydrate	41.4g
sugar, total	7.5g
Fibre – NSP	2.7g
Sodium	51.6mg

—— COOK'S TIP ——

For risotto with an even creamier taste,
bring the wine and water to a simmer in
a separate saucepan, and then add to the
rice a ladleful at a time, allowing each
quantity of liquid to be absorbed before
adding the next.

Roast Vegetables with Artichokes

A colourful medley of vegetables
perfect for winter evenings.

INGREDIENTS

Serves 4
2 × 400g/14oz cans artichoke hearts

2 × 400g/14oz cans broad beans
60ml/4 tbsp olive oil

4 turnips, peeled and sliced thickly, or
scrubbed and left whole

4 medium carrots, scrubbed and
left whole

4 leeks, sliced thickly

2 large courgettes, chopped into large
chunks or 4 small courgettes wiped,
topped and tailed, and left whole

90g/3½oz fresh spinach or frozen
spinach leaf, defrosted

30ml/2 tbsp pumpkin seeds

15ml/1 tbsp mushroom ketchup

ground black pepper

rice or baked potatoes, to serve (optional)

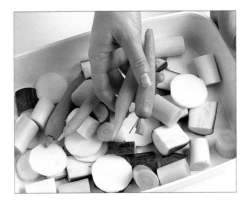

1 Preheat the oven to 180°C/350°F/
Gas 4. Drain the artichoke hearts
and broad beans. Put the olive oil in
the bottom of an ovenproof dish, then
add all the other ingredients apart from
the mushroom ketchup, pumpkin seeds
and black pepper.

2 Cover the dish, then cook the
vegetables for 30–40 minutes or
until the turnips are soft.

3 Add the pumpkin seeds, mushroom
ketchup and pepper. Serve alone or
with rice or baked potatoes.

—— COOK'S TIP ——

If you are in a hurry, cook the vegetables in
a microwave on high for 4 minutes, then
transfer to the oven for 20 minutes.

—— NUTRITION NOTES ——

Per portion:

Energy	373kcals/1529kJ
Fat, total	13.7g
saturated fat	2.1g
Protein	24.1g
Carbohydrate	43.0g
sugar, total	15.7g
Fibre – NSP	16.3g
Sodium	657mg

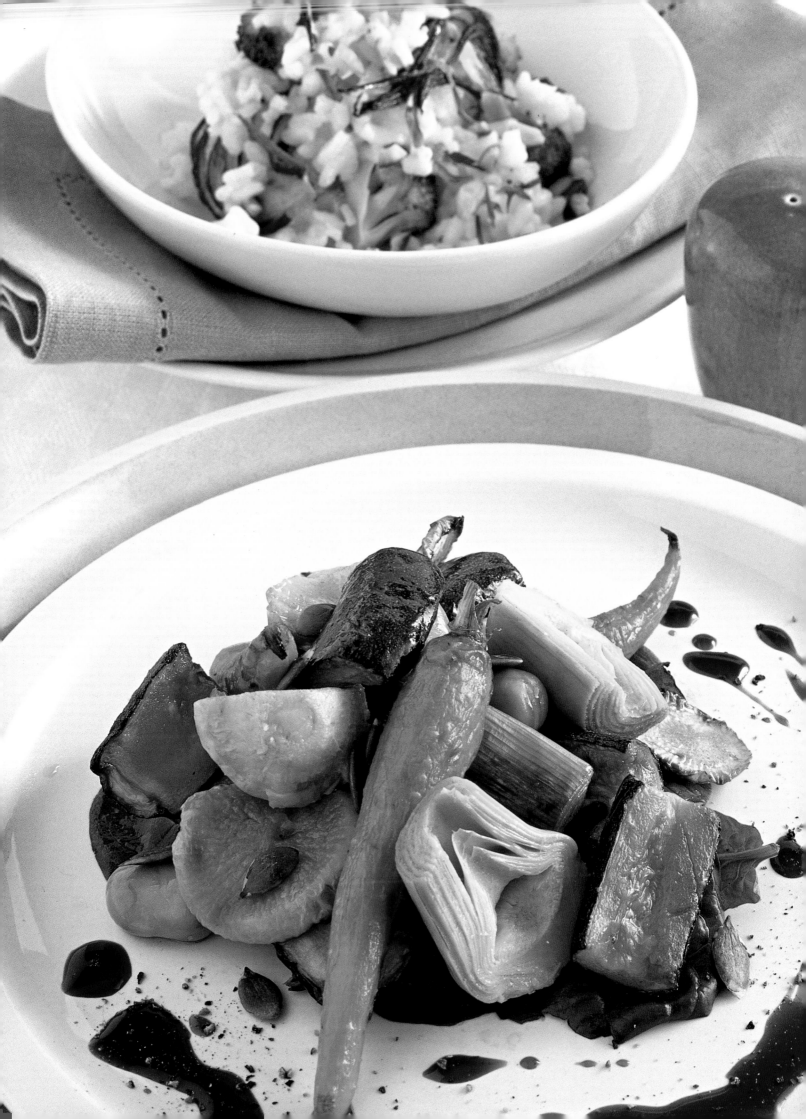

Potato, Leek and Apple Pie

Apples are the unusual ingredient used to flavour this dish. A perfect meal on a cold winter evening.

INGREDIENTS

Serves 6
1.5kg/3lb old potatoes, or, if you are on a solanacae-free diet, sweet potatoes
3 leeks, sliced
60ml/4 tbsp olive oil
3 onions, roughly chopped
small head of celery, chopped
2 large cooking apples,
50g/2oz potato flour or, if you are on a solanacae-free diet, cornflour
450ml/¾ pint/scant 2 cups milk or, if you are on a dairy-free diet, soya milk
75g/3oz pumpkin seeds, partially pulverized in a food processor
15ml/1 tbsp sesame seeds
salt and ground black pepper

1 Preheat the oven to 180°C/350°F/ Gas 4. Scrub the potatoes or sweet potatoes well and cut into thin slices. Par-cook them, with the leeks, in a steamer or microwave for about 10 minutes or until softened.

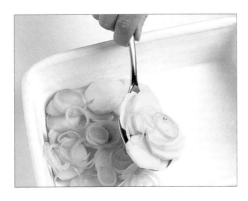

2 Lightly grease a shallow, ovenproof dish. Arrange half of the potatoes and all of the leeks in a layer at the bottom of the dish.

3 Peel, core and dice the apples. Heat 45ml/3 tbsp of the oil in a pan and gently cook the onions, celery and apple until the onion and celery are soft.

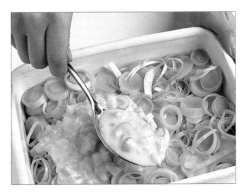

4 Add the potato or cornflour, stir well, then gradually add the milk and continue to cook until the sauce thickens slightly. Spoon this mixture over the potatoes and leeks then cover with the remaining slices of potato.

5 Brush the top of the potatoes with the remaining 15ml/1 tbsp oil. Season, then sprinkle over the pumpkin and sesame seeds.

6 Bake for 20–30 minutes or until the dish is well heated through and the potatoes on top are lightly browned. Serve at once.

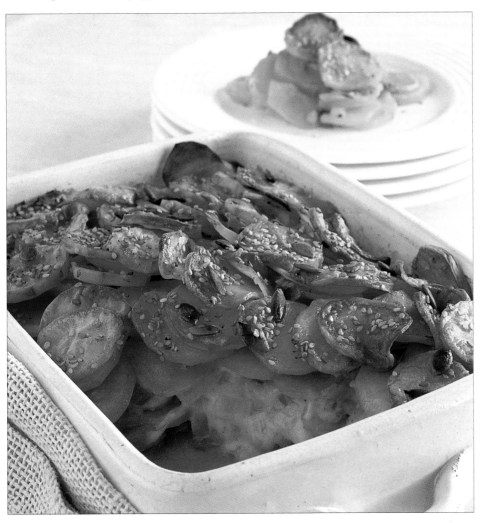

COOK'S TIP

If you have trouble slicing the potatoes or sweet potatoes, cook them whole and slice them when cooked.

NUTRITION NOTES

Per portion:

Energy	446kcals/1827kJ
Fat, total	15.1g
saturated fat	7.1g
Protein	12.4g
Carbohydrate	69.1g
sugar, total	16.2g
Fibre – NSP	6.6g
Sodium	69.7mg

Buckwheat Pancakes with Mushroom Sauce

These pancakes are very adaptable and can be used with sweet fillings as well as savoury.

INGREDIENTS

Serves 4

115g/4oz/1 cup buckwheat flour
1 large egg
120ml/4fl oz/½ cup water
150ml/¼ pint/⅔ cup milk or, if you are
  on a dairy-free diet, soya milk
30ml/2 tbsp olive oil
2 medium leeks, wiped and sliced
1 clove garlic, finely chopped, or 5ml/
  1 tsp puréed garlic
200g/7oz button mushrooms, wiped
  and sliced
15ml/1 tbsp potato flour or, if you are
  on a solanacae-free diet, cornflour
450ml/¾ pint/scant 2 cups milk or,
  if you are on a dairy-free diet,
  unsweetened soya milk
30ml/2 tbsp sweetcorn (tinned or
  frozen will do fine)
50g/2oz chopped toasted hazelnuts
salt and ground black pepper
chopped fresh parsley, to garnish

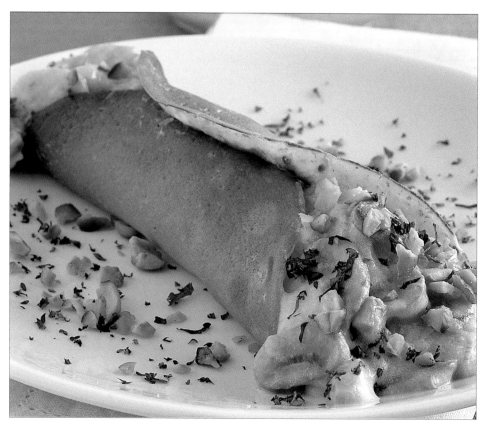

1 To make the pancakes, whizz the flour, egg, water, milk and a pinch of salt in a food processor, then allow the mixture to stand for 10–15 minutes.

2 Heat a pancake pan with a tiny dribble of oil. Pour one small ladleful of the mixture into the pan and cook quickly on both sides. The pancakes should be quite thin and you should get eight out of the mixture. Reserve half of the pancakes to use later, perhaps for pudding. Set them aside with a layer of clear film or greaseproof paper between each one.

3 To make the filling for the pancakes, heat the olive oil in a shallow pan and cook the leeks and garlic until just beginning to soften. Add the mushrooms and continue to cook briskly till the mushrooms are done and their juices running.

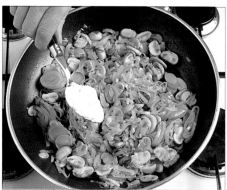

4 Add the potato or cornflour off the heat, stir well, then gradually add the milk and stir until the sauce is quite smooth. Return to the heat and continue to stir until the sauce thickens.

5 Add the sweetcorn and hazelnuts and cook for 2–3 minutes to allow the flavours to amalgamate. Season.

6 Fill each pancake with a spoonful of the filling (reserving some for later). Fold the pancakes over and arrange them in an ovenproof, non-metallic dish.

7 Cover with clear film and reheat in a microwave on full power for 2–3 minutes. Alternatively, cover with foil and reheat in the oven at 180°C/ 350°F/Gas 4 for about 30 minutes. Reheat the remaining sauce and serve it with the pancakes. Sprinkle with parsley and serve.

COOK'S TIP

If filling the pancakes is fiddly, place them in a dish and alternate with layers of the sauce.

NUTRITION NOTES

Per portion:

Energy	480kcals/1967kJ
Fat, total	18.6g
saturated fat	3.3g
Protein	15.1g
Carbohydrate	66.2g
sugar, total	9.0g
Fibre – NSP	2.3g
Sodium	135mg

Green Lentils with Beans and Sun-dried Tomatoes

Although this dish can be eaten immediately, the flavour improves if left to "rest" for 24 hours. Reheat well before serving.

INGREDIENTS

Serves 4
60ml/4 tbsp olive oil
4 medium leeks, finely sliced
2 large courgettes, finely diced
50g/2oz sun-dried tomatoes, chopped in large pieces or, if you are on a solanacae-free diet, 50g/2oz chopped black olives
150g/5oz/¾ cup green lentils
200ml/7fl oz/scant 1 cup Retsina or dry white wine
400ml/14fl oz/1⅔ cups water
16 string beans, chopped roughly
soy sauce, which should be tamari if you are on a wheat-free diet
chopped fresh flat leaf parsley

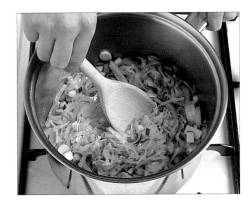

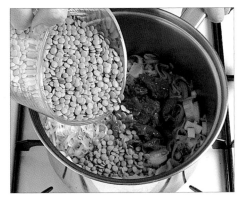

1 Heat the oil in a pan and sweat the leeks and courgettes, covered, for 15–20 minutes or until the vegetables are well softened.

2 Add the sun-dried tomatoes, if using, the green lentils and the wine and water.

3 Bring back to a simmer, cover and cook for 20–30 minutes or until the lentils are cooked.

COOK'S TIP

This is a good dish to make in a table-top cooker or electric frying pan if you find it easier. It can be cooked in and served from the same pan.

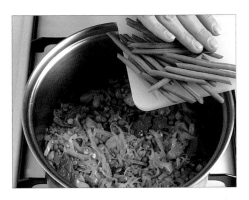

4 Add the string beans and the chopped black olives, if using, to the pan and continue to cook for a further 5–10 minutes, until the beans are tender but not soft.

5 Season with soy sauce and sprinkle with parsley just before serving.

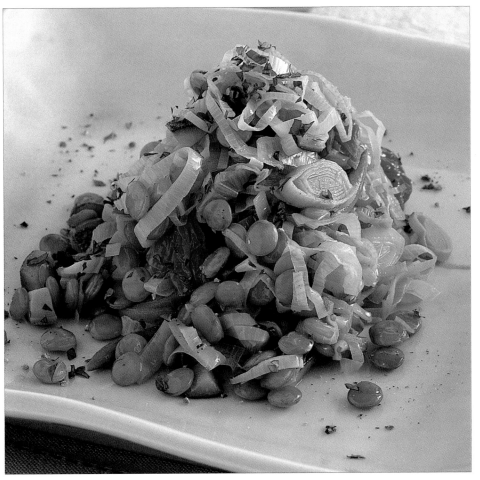

NUTRITION NOTES

Per portion:

Energy	338kcals/1385kJ
Fat, total	18.8g
saturated fat	2.6g
Protein	12.3g
Carbohydrate	23.3g
sugar, total	4.4g
Fibre – NSP	6.1g
Sodium	133mg

Provençal Chard Omelette

This traditional flat omelette can also be made with fresh spinach, but chard leaves are typical in Provence. It is delicious served with small black Niçoise olives.

INGREDIENTS

Serves 6

675g/1½lb chard leaves without stalks
60ml/4 tbsp olive oil
large onion, sliced or 30ml/2 tbsp
   dried onion
2 eggs
salt and ground black pepper
sprig of fresh parsley, to garnish

1 Wash the chard well in several changes of water and pat dry. Stack four or five leaves at a time and slice across into thin ribbons (you can do this with scissors). Steam the chard until wilted, then drain in a sieve and press out any liquid with the back of a spoon.

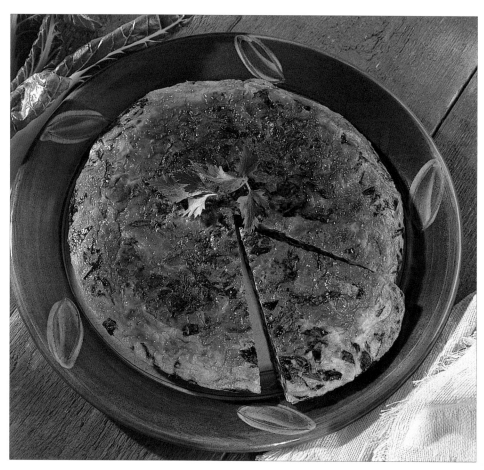

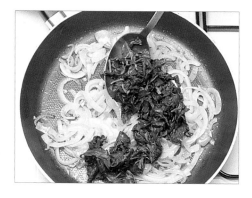

2 Heat 30ml/2 tbsp of the olive oil in a large frying pan. Add the onion and cook over a medium-low heat for about 10 minutes until soft, stirring occasionally. Add the chard and cook for a further 2–4 minutes until the leaves are tender.

COOK'S TIP

If you prefer, you can put the pan under a grill to cook the top – or just cook the whole thing on the hob for slightly longer at a lower heat, then serve it from the pan.

---

3 In a large bowl, beat the eggs and season with salt and pepper, then stir in the cooked vegetables.

4 Heat the remaining 30ml/2 tbsp oil in a large non-stick frying pan over a medium-high heat. Pour in the egg mixture and reduce the heat to medium-low. Cook the omelette, covered, for 5–7 minutes, or until the egg mixture is set around the edges and almost set on top.

NUTRITION NOTES

Per portion:

Energy	135kcals/553kJ
Fat, total	10.3g
saturated fat	1.7g
Protein	5.9g
Carbohydrate	5.0g
sugar, total	3.9g
Fibre – NSP	2.9g
Sodium	185mg

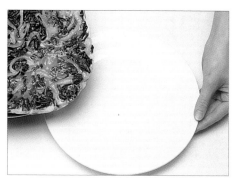

5 To turn the omelette over, loosen around the edges with a palette knife and gently slide it on to a large plate. Place the frying pan over the omelette and, holding them tightly, carefully invert the pan and plate together. Lift off the plate and continue to cook the omelette for a further 2–3 minutes.

6 Slide the omelette on to a serving plate and serve hot or at room temperature, cut into wedges and garnished with a sprig of fresh parsley.

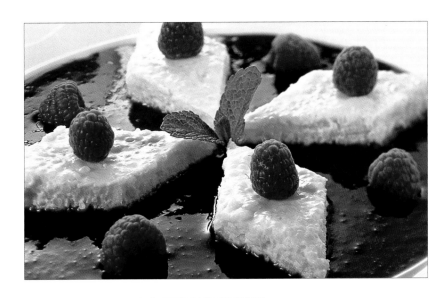

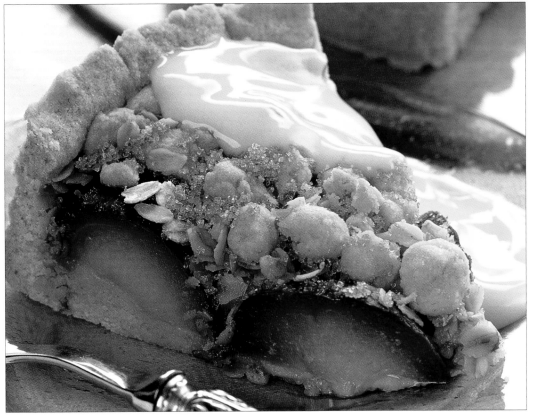

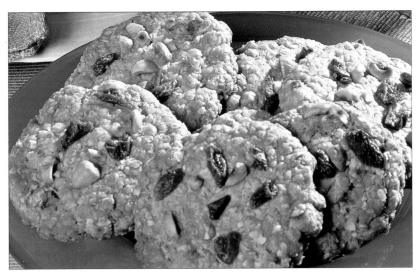

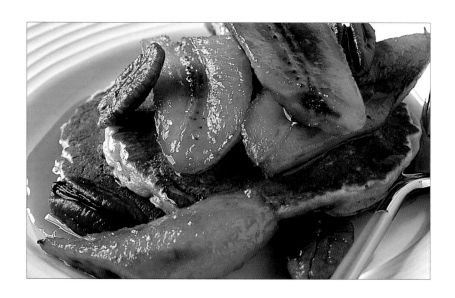

DESSERTS AND BAKING

This selection of delicious cakes and breads is suitable not just for an

arthritic diet but for wheat- and dairy-free diets as well. Try the

delicious Coconut Cream Dessert or Plum Crumble Pie for a rich

treat, or one of the three recipes based on fresh fruit for a more simple

dessert. The Courgette and Double-ginger Cake is a must for

arthritis sufferers, as ginger can reduce inflammation in some people.

The breads are good, too; slice thickly and serve with honey or jam.

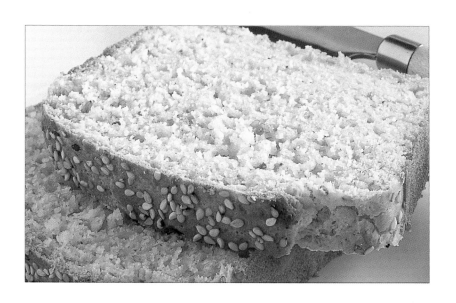

Oaty Pancakes with Caramel Bananas

INGREDIENTS

Makes 10

75g/3oz/⅔ cup unbleached plain flour, sifted or, if you are on a wheat-free diet, rice flour

50g/2oz/½ cup wholemeal flour or, if you are on a wheat-free diet, chick-pea flour

50g/2oz/½ cup porridge oats

5ml/1 tsp baking powder, wheat-free if you are on a wheat-free diet

pinch of salt

5ml/1 tsp golden caster sugar

1 egg

15ml/1 tbsp sunflower oil, plus extra for frying

250ml/8fl oz/1 cup semi-skimmed milk or, if you are on a dairy-free diet, soya, rice or coconut milk

For the caramel bananas

25g/1oz/2 tbsp butter or sunflower oil if you are on a dairy-free diet

15ml/1 tbsp maple syrup

3 ripe bananas, halved and quartered lengthways

25g/1oz/¼ cup pecan nuts

1 Firstly, make the pancakes. Place the flours, oats, baking powder, salt and sugar in a large mixing bowl and stir them together.

2 Make a well in the centre of the flour mixture and add the egg, sunflower oil and about a quarter of the milk.

3 Use a hand-held whisk to mix the ingredients well, then gradually add the rest of the milk to make a thick batter. Leave to rest for 20 minutes in the fridge.

— NUTRITION NOTES —	
Per portion:	
Energy	148kcals/606kJ
Fat, total	5.5g
saturated fat	1.9g
Protein	4.0g
Carbohydrate	22.0g
sugar, total	8.7g
Fibre – NSP	1.4g
Sodium	42.9mg

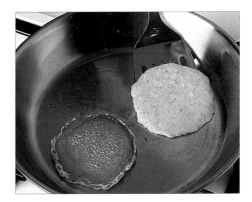

4 Heat a large, lightly oiled frying pan. Using about 30ml/2 tbsp of batter for each pancake, cook two or three pancakes at a time. Cook for 3 minutes on each side or until golden. Keep warm while you cook the remaining seven or eight pancakes.

5 To make the caramel bananas, wipe out the frying pan and add the butter or oil. Heat gently, then add the maple syrup and stir well. Add the bananas and pecan nuts to the pan.

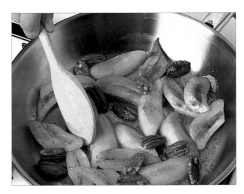

6 Allow to cook, covered, for about 4 minutes, turning once, or until the bananas have just softened and the sauce has caramelized slightly. To serve, place two pancakes on each of five warm plates and top with the bananas and pecan nuts. Serve immediately.

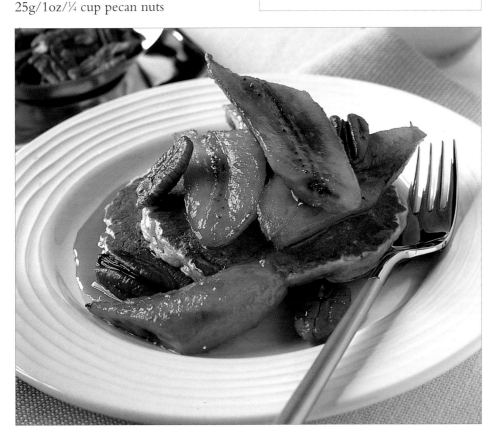

— HEALTH BENEFITS —

Bananas are an excellent source of energy, and they also contain potassium, which is essential for the healthy functioning of all the cells in our bodies.

Plum Crumble Pie

Polenta adds a wonderful golden hue and crunchiness to the crumble topping on this fruit-filled pie. Plums are a rich source of the antioxidant, vitamin E.

INGREDIENTS

Serves 6

115g/4oz/1 cup unbleached plain
   flour, sifted or, if you are on a wheat-
   free diet, rice flour
115g/4oz/1 cup wholemeal flour or,
   if you are on a wheat-free diet,
   chick-pea flour
150g/5oz/¾ cup golden caster sugar
115g/4oz/1 cup polenta
5ml/1 tsp baking powder, wheat-free if
   you are on a wheat-free diet
pinch of salt
150g/5oz/10 tbsp butter or, if you are
   on a dairy-free diet, dairy-free spread,
   plus extra for greasing
1 egg
15ml/1 tbsp olive oil
25g/1oz/¼ cup rolled oats
15ml/1 tbsp demerara sugar
custard or cream, to serve (optional)

For the filling
10ml/2 tsp caster sugar
15ml/1 tbsp polenta
450g/1lb dark plums

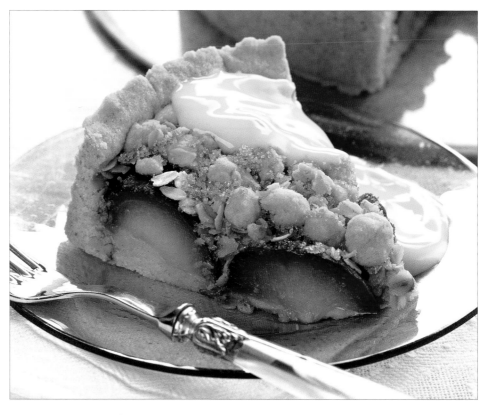

1 Mix together the flours, sugar, polenta, baking powder and salt in a large bowl. Rub in the butter or spread with your fingers until the mixture resembles fine breadcrumbs. Stir in the egg and olive oil and enough cold water to form a smooth dough.

2 Grease a 23cm/9in spring-form cake tin. Press two-thirds of the dough evenly over the base and up the sides of the tin. Wrap the remaining dough in clear film and chill while you make the filling.

3 Preheat the oven to 180°C/350°F/ Gas 4. Sprinkle the sugar and polenta into the pastry case.

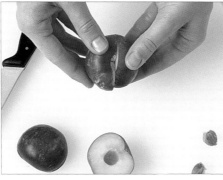

4 Using a sharp knife, cut the plums in half and remove the stones. Place the plums, cut-side down, on top of the polenta dough.

--- NUTRITION NOTES ---

Per portion:

Energy	535kcals/2193kJ
Fat, total	24.3g
saturated fat	14.3g
Protein	7.0g
Carbohydrate	75.3g
sugar, total	33.4g
Fibre – NSP	3.0g
Sodium	208mg

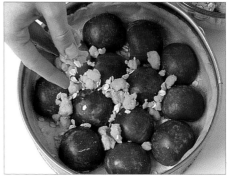

5 Remove the remaining dough from the fridge and crumble it between your fingers, then combine with the oats. Sprinkle evenly over the plums, then sprinkle with demerara sugar.

6 Bake for 50 minutes or until golden. Leave for 15 minutes. Remove the sides of the cake tin and slide the base on to a serving dish. Serve with custard or cream, if liked.

--- COOK'S TIP ---

The polenta dough can be made in a food processor if you find it easier.

Three Simple Fruit Desserts

Fresh Pineapple with Kirsch

Ingredients

Serves 6
1 large pineapple
30ml/2 tbsp caster sugar
15ml/3 tsp Kirsch or cherry brandy
mint sprigs, to decorate

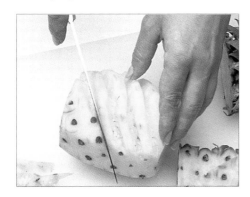

1 Using a large sharp knife, cut off the top and bottom of the pineapple. Cut off the peel from top to bottom and then remove the eyes, cutting in a V-shaped wedge.

2 Cut the pineapple into slices. Use an apple corer to remove the tough central core, if you like. Arrange the pineapple slices on a serving plate. Sprinkle evenly with sugar and Kirsch or cherry brandy. Chill until ready to serve, then decorate with mint sprigs.

Cook's tip

Pineapple can be quite tricky to peel, so use tinned pineapple if your hands are arthritic.

Nutrition Notes

Per portion:

Energy	46.5kcals/190kJ
Fat, total	0.0g
saturated fat	0.0g
Protein	0.2g
Carbohydrate	10.7g
sugar, total	10.7g
Fibre – NSP	0.5g
Sodium	1.0mg

Melon with Raspberries

Ingredients

Serves 2
2 tiny or 1 small ripe melon
115g/4oz/1 cup fresh raspberries
15–30ml/1–2 tbsp raspberry
  liqueur (optional)

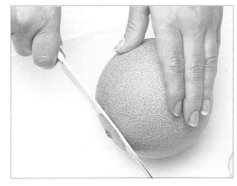

1 Cut off a thin slice from the bottom of each melon to create a stable base. If the melons are tiny, cut off the top third and scoop out as much of the flesh as possible from each top. Cut the flesh into tiny dice.

2 If a larger melon is used, cut off a thin slice from both the top and bottom to create two stable bases; then split the melon in half and dice the flesh. In either case, scoop out and discard the seeds.

3 Fill the centre of the melon halves with any diced melon and the raspberries and, if you like, sprinkle with a little liqueur. Chill before serving or serve on a bed of crushed ice.

Nutrition Notes

Per portion:

Energy	46kcals/188kJ
Fat, total	0.3g
saturated fat	0.0g
Protein	1.4g
Carbohydrate	10.2g
sugar, total	10.2g
Fibre – NSP	2.0g
Sodium	43mg

Grilled Fruit Kebabs

Ingredients

Makes 6
4 or 5 kinds of firm ripe fruit, such as
  grapes, pear and nectarine slices,
  mango and pineapple cubes and
  tangerine segments
25g/1oz/2 tbsp walnut oil
grated rind and juice of 1 orange, or
  omit if you are on a citrus-free diet
sugar, to taste
pinch of ground cinnamon or nutmeg
yogurt, soured cream, crème fraîche,
  soya cream or fruit coulis, to serve

1 Preheat the grill and line a baking sheet with foil.

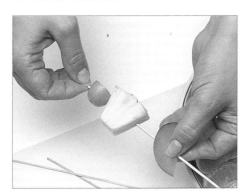

2 Thread the fruit on to six skewers (dampened if wood), alternating fruits to create an attractive pattern. Place on the foil and brush with oil. Spoon over the orange rind and juice, if using, and sprinkle with the sugar and spice. Grill for 2–3 minutes until the sugar just begins to caramelize. Serve immediately, with your chosen topping.

Nutrition Notes

Per portion:

Energy	57kcals/233kJ
Fat, total	3.6g
saturated fat	0.3g
Protein	0.3g
Carbohydrate	6.0g
sugar, total	6.0g
Fibre – NSP	0.8g
Sodium	2.5mg

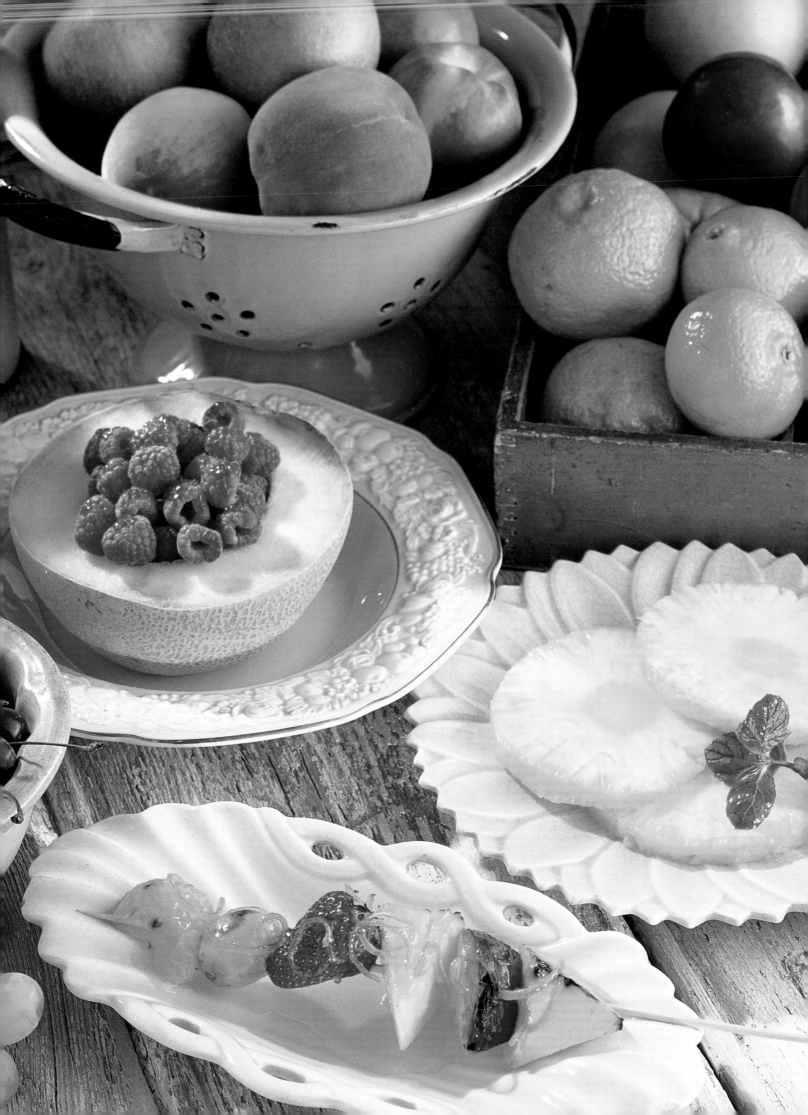

Coconut Cream Dessert

The soft, sticky texture of Thai fragrant rice makes it perfect for this dish. Desserts such as these are served in countries all over the Far East, often with mangoes, pineapple or guavas.

INGREDIENTS

Serves 4

75g/3oz/scant ½ cup Thai fragrant rice, soaked overnight in 175ml/ 6fl oz/¾ cup water
350ml/12fl oz/1½ cups coconut milk
150ml/¼ pint/⅔ cup coconut cream
50g/2oz/¼ cup caster sugar
fresh raspberries and mint leaves, to decorate

For the coulis

75g/3oz/¾ cup blackcurrants, stalks removed
30ml/2 tbsp caster sugar
75g/3oz/½ cup raspberries, thawed if frozen

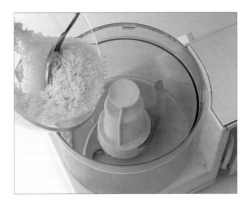

1 Put the Thai fragrant rice and its soaking water into a food processor and process for a few minutes until the mixture is soupy.

2 Heat the coconut milk and cream in a non-stick saucepan. When the mixture is on the point of boiling, stir in the rice mixture. Cook very gently for 10 minutes, stirring constantly, then stir in the sugar and continue cooking for 10–15 minutes more, or until the mixture is thick and creamy.

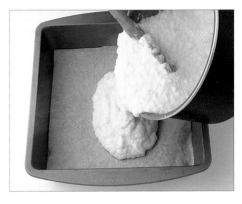

3 Pour the rice mixture into a shallow baking tin that has been lined with non-stick baking paper. Cool, then chill until firm.

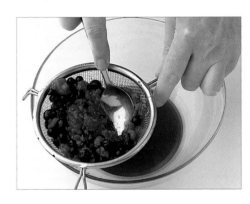

4 To make the coulis, put the blackcurrants in a bowl. Sprinkle with sugar and set aside for 30 minutes. Tip into a sieve with the raspberries. Press the fruit through the sieve into a bowl. Add sugar to taste.

5 Cut the rice mixture into diamonds. Spoon the coulis on to each plate, arrange the diamonds on top and decorate with raspberries and mint.

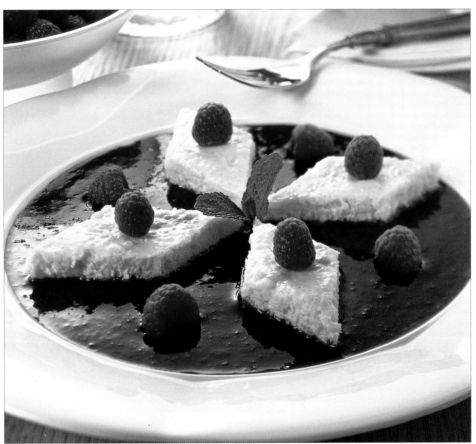

NUTRITION NOTES	
Per portion:	
Energy	169kcals/692kJ
Fat, total	0.5g
saturated fat	0.2g
Protein	1.9g
Carbohydrate	42.9g
sugar, total	26.6g
Fibre – NSP	1.2g
Sodium	104mg

Courgette and Double-ginger Cake

Both fresh and preserved ginger are used to flavour this unusual tea bread. It is delicious served warm, cut into thick slices and spread with butter or jam.

INGREDIENTS

Serves 10

3 eggs
225g/8oz/generous 1 cup caster sugar
250ml/8fl oz/1 cup sunflower oil
5ml/1 tsp vanilla essence
15ml/1 tbsp syrup from a jar of
    stem ginger
225g/8oz courgettes, grated
2.5cm/1in piece fresh root ginger,
    grated or 5ml/1 tsp puréed ginger or
    7.5ml/1½ tsp ground ginger
350g/12oz/3 cups unbleached plain
    flour or, if you are on a wheat-free
    diet, 150g/5oz/¾ cup rice flour and
    200g/7oz/2¼ cups pulverized oats
5ml/1 tsp baking powder, wheat-free,
    if you are on a wheat-free diet
5ml/1 tsp ground cinnamon
pinch of salt
2 pieces stem ginger, chopped
15ml/1 tbsp demerara sugar

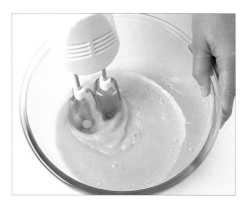

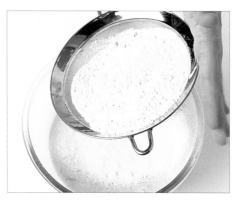

1 Preheat the oven to 190°C/375°F/ Gas 5. In a large bowl, beat together the eggs and sugar until light and fluffy. Slowly beat in the oil until the mixture forms a batter. Mix in the vanilla essence and ginger syrup, then stir in the courgettes and fresh, puréed or ground ginger.

2 Sift the flour (or rice flour and oats), baking powder, cinnamon and salt into the batter. Fold the dry ingredients into the courgette mixture.

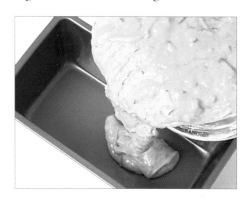

HEALTH BENEFITS

• Ginger has many beneficial attributes, not least of which is its ability to block the enzymes that lead to inflammation.
• Courgettes are a good source of betacarotene, vitamin C and folate.

3 Lightly grease a 900g/2lb loaf tin and pour in the courgette mixture. Smooth and level the top, then sprinkle the chopped ginger and demerara sugar over the surface.

4 Bake for 1 hour until a skewer inserted into the centre comes out clean. Leave the cake in the tin to cool for about 20 minutes, then turn out on to a wire rack.

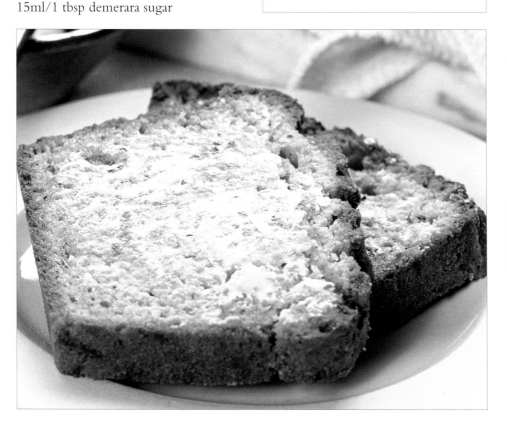

NUTRITION NOTES

Per portion:

Energy	393kcals/1611kJ
Fat, total	19.8g
saturated fat	3.11g
Protein	5.7g
Carbohydrate	51.2g
sugar, total	24.5g
Fibre – NSP	1.3g
Sodium	25mg

Apricot and Hazelnut Oat Cookies

These cookie-cum-flapjacks have a chewy, crumbly texture. They are sprinkled with apricots and toasted hazelnuts, but any combination of dried fruit and nuts can be used.

INGREDIENTS

Makes 9

115g/4oz/1 cup self-raising flour, sifted or, if you are on a wheat-free diet, 115g/4oz/1 cup rice flour plus 10ml/2 tsp wheat-free baking powder
115g/4oz/1 cup porridge oats
75g/3oz/scant ½ cup chopped ready-to-eat dried unsulphured apricots
115g/4oz/½ cup unsalted butter, or dairy-free spread if you are on a dairy-free diet, plus extra for greasing
75g/3oz/scant ½ cup golden caster sugar
15ml/1 tbsp clear honey

For the topping

25g/1oz/2 tbsp chopped ready-to-eat dried unsulphured apricots
25g/1oz/¼ cup toasted and chopped hazelnuts

1 Preheat the oven to 160°C/325°F/ Gas 3. Lightly grease a large baking sheet. Place the flour (or rice flour and baking powder), oats and chopped apricots in a large mixing bowl.

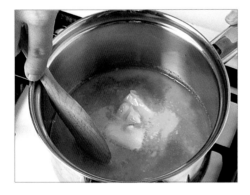

2 Put the butter or dairy-free spread, sugar and honey in a saucepan and cook over a gentle heat, until the butter melts and the sugar dissolves, stirring the mixture occasionally. Remove the pan from the heat.

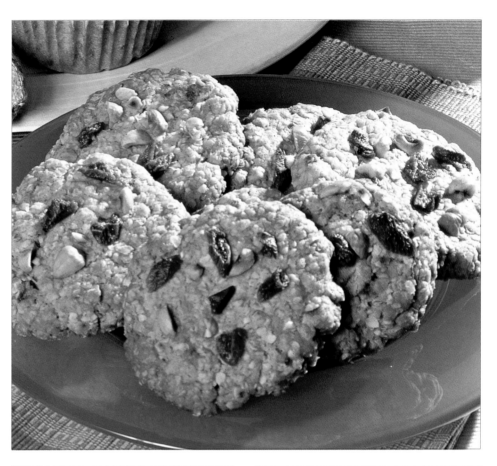

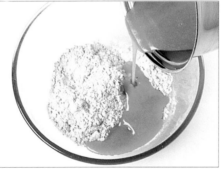

3 Pour the honey and sugar mixture into the bowl containing the flour, oats and apricots. Mix well with a wooden spoon to form a sticky dough. Divide the dough into nine pieces and place on the prepared baking sheet. Press into 1cm/½in thick rounds.

4 Scatter over the topping of apricots and hazelnuts and press into the dough. Bake the cookies for about 15 minutes, until they are golden and slightly crisp. Leave to cool on the baking sheet for 5 minutes, then transfer to a wire rack.

COOK'S TIP

Dried fruit such as apricots are easier to chop if you use scissors rather than a knife.

NUTRITION NOTES

Per portion:

Energy	276kcals/1130kJ
Fat, total	11.9g
saturated fat	7.0g
Protein	4.4g
Carbohydrate	39.7g
sugar, total	11.7g
Fibre – NSP	2.4g
Sodium	104mg

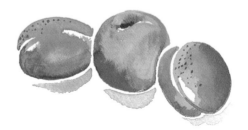

Wheat-free Brown Bread

This is a good bread if you are avoiding wheat and dairy products. It is similar in taste and texture to a fairly dense wholemeal wheaten loaf.

INGREDIENTS

Makes 1 loaf
350g/12oz/3 cups brown rice flour
50g/2oz/½ cup buckwheat flour
50g/2oz/½ cup potato flour or
   cornflour
5ml/1 tsp soya flour
2.5ml/½ tsp salt
10ml/2 tsp sugar
7.5ml/1½ tsp cream of tartar
1.5ml/¼ tsp bicarbonate of soda
10ml/2 tsp easy-bake yeast
20g/¾oz butter or, if you are on a
   dairy-free diet, dairy-free spread
1 egg
15ml/1 tbsp sesame seeds (optional)

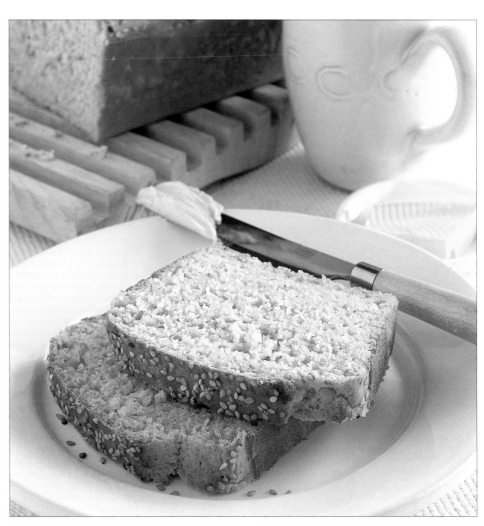

1 Preheat the oven to 180°C/350°F/ Gas 4. Grease a loaf tin or a round cake tin. Place all of the flours, the salt, sugar, cream of tartar, bicarbonate of soda and yeast in a large mixing bowl. Mix thoroughly.

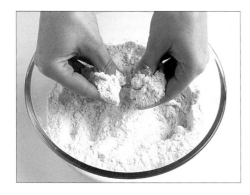

2 Rub in the butter or spread, then stir in the egg and half the sesame seeds, if you are using them.

3 Make up 425ml/¾ pint/2 cups warm water with 150ml/¼ pint/ ⅔ cup boiling water, cooled with 275ml/½ pint/1⅓ cups tap water. Stir this into the other ingredients.

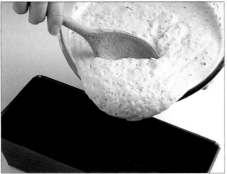

4 Pour the mixture into the prepared tin. Sprinkle with the remaining sesame seeds, if using. Bake for about 40 minutes, or until the bread is risen and a skewer comes out clean.

5 Cool in the tin for 5–10 minutes under a dish towel, then carefully knock out the bread on to a wire rack. Cover with a dish towel and leave until quite cold before cutting.

COOK'S TIP

• The uncooked mixture will be very runny but it will firm up during baking to produce a moist but compact loaf.
• If your hands are stiff you may find it easier to mix all of the ingredients together in a food processor.

NUTRITION NOTES

Per loaf:

Energy	1855kcals/7728kJ
Fat, total	26.5g
saturated fat	12.7g
Protein	38.1g
Carbohydrate	36.0g
sugar, total	1.5g
Fibre – NSP	10.9g
Sodium	1245mg

Rice Flour and Banana Bread

This is a great bread for those trying to avoid wheat and dairy products. It has more of the texture of a cake than of bread, but still tastes pretty "bready". It is delicious warm, served with jam or honey.

INGREDIENTS

Makes 1 loaf

2 bananas

150g/5oz rice flour

50g/2oz sunflower spread

10ml/2 tsp baking powder, wheat-free if you are on a wheat-free diet

1 egg

100ml/3½fl oz/½ cup milk or, if you are on a dairy-free diet, soya milk

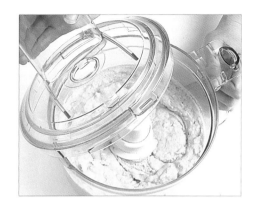

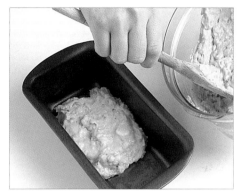

1 Place all of the ingredients for the bread in a food processor and purée until smooth. You can also use a hand-held blender in a bowl if you prefer. Meanwhile preheat the oven to 180°C/350°F/Gas 4 and lightly grease a small loaf tin.

2 Spoon the mixture into the tin and bake for 35 minutes or until a skewer comes out clean.

3 Remove from the oven and allow to cool slightly. Knock out of the tin and place on a wire rack to cool, covered in a dish towel.

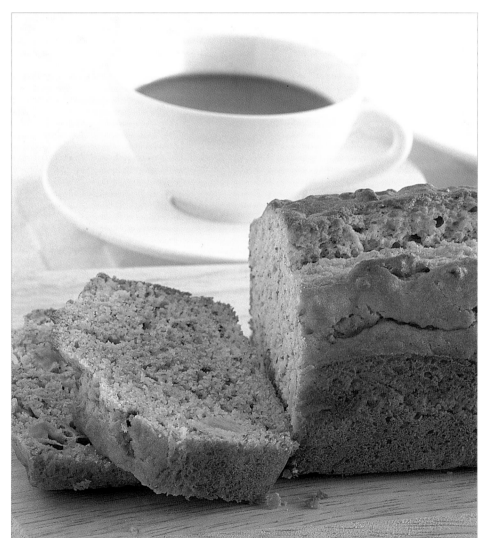

COOK'S TIP

You could easily turn this bread into a cake by adding 45ml/3 tbsp demerara sugar when you purée the bananas, and stirring in 30ml/2 tbsp plump raisins or other dried fruit before it goes into the oven.

NUTRITION NOTES

Per loaf:

Energy	1236kcals/5067kJ
Fat, total	50.4g
saturated fat	15.3g
Protein	22.4g
Carbohydrate	172g
sugar, total	47g
Fibre – NSP	5.2g
Sodium	544mg

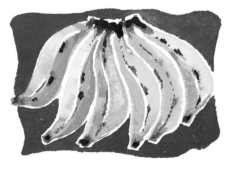

INFORMATION FILE

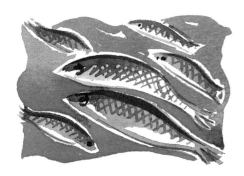

USEFUL ADDRESSES

Arthritis Care
18 Stephenson Way
London NW1 2HD
Tel: 020 7916 1500
www.arthritiscare.org.uk
Helpline: 0845 600 6868 (open 24 hours)

Arthritis Research Campaign
Copeman House, St Mary's Court
St Mary's Gate
Chesterfield
Derbyshire S41 7TD
Tel: 01246 558033

DIALs
Disabled Information and Advice Lines
DIAL UK
Park Lodge, St Catherine's Hospital
Tickhill Road
Doncaster DN4 8QN
Tel: 01302 310 123
Check your telephone book for list of
local DIALs

**Institute for Complementary
Medicine**
PO Box 194
Tavery Quay
London SE16 1QZ
Tel: 020 7237 5165
List of qualified practitioners available (send
large sae and state therapy)

Disabled Living Foundation
380–384 Harrow Road
London W9 2HU
Tel: 020 7289 6111

RADAR
The Royal Association for Disability and
Rehabilitation
Unit 12, City Forum
250 City Road
London EC1V 8AF
Tel: 020 7250 3222

Northern Ireland
Disability Action
2 Annadale Avenue
Belfast BT7 3JH
Tel: 028 9049 1011

Scotland
Disability Scotland
Princes House
5 Shandwick Place
Edinburgh EH2 4RG
Tel: 0131 229 8632

Wales
Disability Wales
'Llys Ifor' Crescent Road
Caerfilly CF 83 1XL
Tel: 029 2088 7325

Children
**Children's Chronic Arthritis
Association**
47 Battenhall Avenue
Wocester WR5 2HN
Tel: 029 2088 7325

Equipment
Homecraft/Chestercare
Sidings Road
Lowmoor Road Industrial Estate
Kirkby in Ashfield
Nottinghamshire NG17 7JZ
Tel: 01623 754b047
www.snrehab.com
Mail order aids for every kind of disability

Disabled Living Centres Council
Redbank House
Manchester M8 8QA
Tel: 0161 834 1044
Demonstration and resource centres
throughout the country

AUSTRALIA

The Arthritis Foundation of NSW
Locked Bag 16
PO Box North Parramatta NSW 2151
13 Harold Street
North Parramatta NSW 2151
Tel: 02 9683 1622
email: info@arthritisnsw.org.au
Contact for information on Support Groups

**The Arthritis Foundation of
Victoria Inc**
P O Box 130
Caulfield South
3162 Victoria
Tel: 03 9530 0255

The Arthritis Foundation of Australia
52 Parramatta Road,
Forest Lodge NSW 2037
Tel: 0061 02 9552 6085
Freecall: 1800 011 041

GLOSSARY

ALA (alpha linolenic acid) − an essential
fatty acid, found in oily fish, helpful in
minimizing inflammation

antioxidants − nutrients or enzymes
which neutralize free radicals in the body

cartilage − the protective cushion which
separates bones at the point that they
meet in joints

free radicals − a chemical reaction that
causes damage to the body's tissues

GLAs (gamma linolenic acid) − an
essential fatty acid, found in some seeds,
helpful in minimizing inflammation

NSAIDs (non-steroidal anti-inflammatory
drugs) − drugs that may be prescribed to
help relieve inflammation and pain

prostaglandin − a chemical which can
help to control inflammation

solanacae − a family of foods (potato,
peppers, aubergine and chillies) that may
cause an allergic reaction in some people

synovial fluid − the fluid that lubricates a
joint, allowing it to move freely

INDEX

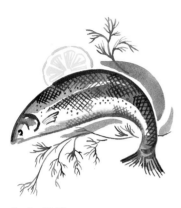

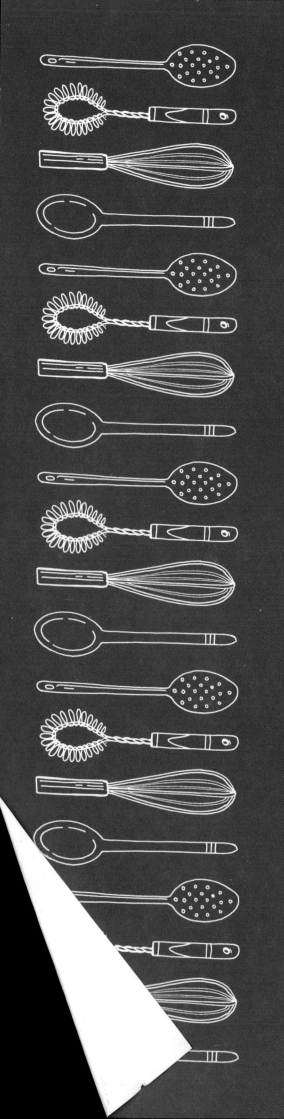